Superfoods for life

Cultured and Fermented
BEVERAGES

Superfoods for life

Cultured and Fermented
BEVERAGES

Meg Thompson

_HEAL DIGESTION
_SUPERCHARGE
 YOUR IMMUNITY
_DETOXIFY YOUR SYSTEM
_75 RECIPES

Fair Winds Press
100 Cummings Center, Suite 406L
Beverly, MA 01915

fairwindspress.com • quarryspoon.com

First published in the USA in 2014 by
Fair Winds Press, a member of
Quarto Publishing Group USA Inc.
100 Cummings Center
Suite 406-L
Beverly, MA 01915-6101
www.fairwindspress.com

Visit www.QuarrySPOON.com and help us celebrate food and culture one spoonful at a time!

18 17 16 15 14   1 2 3 4 5

ISBN: 978-1-59233-601-2

Digital edition published in 2014
eISBN: 978-1-62788-018-3

Library of Congress Cataloging-in-Publication Data available

Cover design by Laura H. Couallier, Laura Herrmann Design
Book layout by Megan Jones Design
Photography by Glenn Scott Photography

Printed and bound in China

The information in this book is for educational purposes only. It is not intended to replace the advice of a physician or medical practitioner. Please see your health care provider before beginning any new health program.

Dedication

For Mat. X

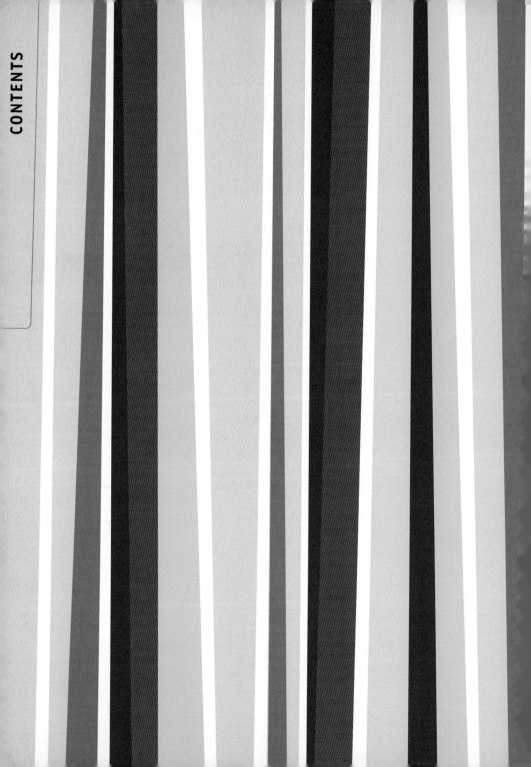

CONTENTS

Cultured and Fermented Beverages

Dear Fermenting Friend,

I am absolutely thrilled to be able to share with you this information on the truly incredible health-giving properties of cultured beverages.

In this book, you will discover that not only do they nourish and heal the digestive system, but also they have other far-reaching benefits, including improving immunity; assisting in detoxification; supporting pregnancy, breast-feeding, and growing children; and fostering radiant skin and a healthy mind. I will also share some trusty naturopathic tonics using fermented herbs to treat basic health conditions. And the best part? They are all so easy and inexpensive to make at home.

When I first began research for this book, I was really excited to share some insights about fermented beverages; however, I wasn't sure how many studies I would find. I knew there were many on gut bacteria and probiotics, but I was less certain about what I would find on fermented beverages. You can imagine how thrilled I was to find dozens of research articles showing the benefits of fermented beverages, in particular kombucha and kefir. They are the heavyweights of the fermented beverage world, and for this reason they receive the lion's share of attention in this book. But please don't dismiss your beet kvass or your sprouted spelt grain rejuvelac—they are just as important as the big kids.

Getting Started: How to Use This Book

Making cultured beverages may seem overwhelming to begin with. The process may not have the sexiness of sourdough, or the mellowness of miso, but making your own fermented beverages is exciting and fun. You just need to find your rhythm. What is not to love about "burping" your turmeric beer, or watching the first bubbles of fermentation form, confirming you have a drink that is truly alive? In fact, at times you may feel like a mad scientist conjuring up experiments. And to be honest, that is what is so fun about making these drinks: You really can create your own brand of specialness with them. Fermenting teaches patience and trust, which is a wonderful thing to have in our homes to keep us grounded.

DID YOU KNOW?

Historically, fermented food and beverages were a part of everyday life. It has only been in relatively recent times, since the introduction of refrigerators and modern preservation methods, that there has been no need for traditional food preservation. Fermenting food improves the longevity of the product and increases its nutrient value. One popular historic example of its use was with Captain James Cook on his voyage to Australia; he fed his crew sauerkraut (fermented cabbage) to prevent them from getting scurvy, which is a disease resulting from a lack of vitamin C. But with modern food preservation methods, we have seen a dramatic reduction in the amount of cultured foods and drinks consumed, while at the same time refined foods have flooded the Western diet. This is not a good combination, especially for our guts, and there are countless health conditions that can be linked back to this general imbalance.

Two of my very favorite things in the world are fermented: coffee and vanilla. A combination of the natural enzymes in the pulp and the yeasts and bacteria from the environment break down the mucilaginous pulp around coffee beans. Vanilla pods are the fermented and dried seedpods of orchids.

Chocolate runs a close third. Chocolate comes from cacao beans, which after harvesting are fermented in vats covered with banana leaves for a few days. So the point I am getting to here is that fermenting is fabulous.

Throughout this book, I discuss various strains and species of the live bacteria found in probiotics. The current expert opinion on probiotics is that we cannot extrapolate and transfer the benefits. For example, if a particular bacteria strain has been shown in research to alleviate eczema, we cannot then say that all probiotics are effective, or even that all species are, but only that one exact strain has been proven to be effective in that research piece. Although I completely respect the research being done and agree that it is necessary to help us understand more about how our bodies interact with bacteria, I feel that this view is a little reductionist. The field of probiotics can be confusing, overwhelming, and expensive. For the average person trying to better his or her heath who is told it is necessary to have this strain for this problem and that strain for that problem, it can all be too much. By taking these strains in isolation, we know how they perform in isolation, but what about taking them in whole foods? I have included as many research articles as I could find using kefir and kombucha, rather than focusing on specific strains, as I feel that is how most people should be consuming their probiotics—as fermented foods and drinks.

There are a couple of ways to go about culturing beverages. The first is by wild fermentation, popularized by Sandor Katz, author of *The Art of Fermentation*. This means relying on the bacteria and yeasts that are naturally present in the food or the environment. The other method is by culturing with the addition of a microbial starter of some kind, like a SCOBY, a packet of yeast, a collection of kefir grains, or whey. I cover both methods in this book.

The final note I want to make is that although this book is full of recipes with exact ingredients, you will most likely get a slightly different result each time you make a particular recipe. The end result of your recipe will depend on the sourness of your cultured beverage to begin with. My advice is to play around with the basic recipes and techniques to get your confidence up, and also to get to know how tart you like your drinks and how long you need to leave them to get that result. Then you can start experimenting!

CHAPTER 1

Fermenting for Healthy Digestion

A healthy gut is essential to the health of our whole body. If our digestive system is not in balance, we may develop not only digestive symptoms but also disease throughout the body.

How do fermented beverages help? They contribute to a healthy gut ecosystem, and they also have specific actions that directly improve its function. Swapping the soda pop for the kombucha, for example, is one simple change that will not only improve digestion, but also make a positive impact on immunity, weight management, energy, and even the way we feel emotionally.

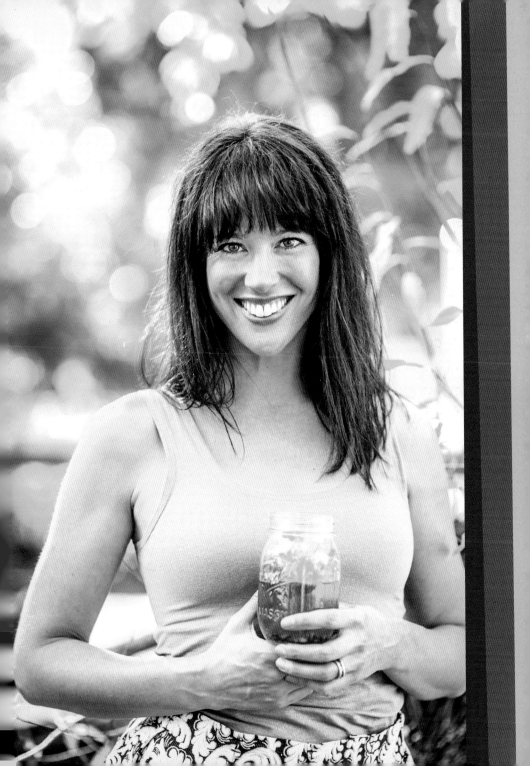

How Does Digestion Work?

Beginning at the mouth, the digestive system involves the liver, gallbladder, pancreas, and colon all working in harmony to keep us functioning well. But digestion starts before food even enters our mouth. We smell something delicious, or we see a fabulous social media feed full of delicious-looking food photos, and they trigger saliva release—they are literally mouthwatering. The release of saliva is controlled by the brain, specifically the autonomic nervous system. Saliva contains an important enzyme, amylase, which initiates the digestion of starch.

Following from this, swallowed food moves through the esophagus into the stomach, where stomach acid is released. Stomach acid and enzymes are the gracious digestive hosts without which the party cannot happen. A reduced production of stomach acid and digestive enzymes leads to problems digesting and absorbing food and nutrients, and it is also associated with a whole host of inflammatory conditions and gastrointestinal infections. The acid not only helps break down protein, but also enhances the bioavailability of minerals and kills off pathogenic bacteria that are harmful to the body. Low stomach acid, or hypochlorhydria, is far more common than over-acidity. Interestingly, it is usually a lack of stomach acid that leads to conditions such as reflux, or gastroesophageal reflux disease (GERD), and not an oversupply of it.

The next step in digestion involves the food being pushed along from the stomach into the small intestine, and at that point juices from the pancreas and liver join the party. This further digests and converts the food into substances that the body can absorb. Absorption of nutrients takes place as food passes through the small intestine. The small intestine is a long tube, about 1 inch (2.5 cm) in diameter and 20 feet (6 meters) in length if stretched out. The tube is lined with finger-like folds called villi. Now imagine every villus is further covered by tiny, hair-like structures called microvilli. Instead of just having the surface area of the tube, it is now increased dramatically with the villi and microvilli to give an actual surface area of roughly 250 square meters—about the size of a tennis court. It is incredible to think that all this is neatly packed up inside us. The villi and microvilli are woven together tightly, and the entire small intestine is further covered in mucus for protection. A strict security system is in place here, and only correctly processed nutrients are absorbed across the barrier into the bloodstream.

After this, waste products from this process move through to the colon, where they are released with a bowel movement for excretion.

But What Makes a Healthy Gut? Bacteria!

Did you know that we have about 2 quarts/2 liters of bacteria lining our digestive tract? These beautiful, hardworking little microbes live protected and nourished by our gut. These microbes outnumber our body cells by a ratio of 10:1, and with ten times more bacteria cells than body cells, it's important to make sure they are well looked after. They are absolutely essential to our health, not only in the digestive system but also in the nervous system and immune system. Every individual has a unique composition of gut bacteria, right from birth. The birthing process itself delivers each child with a dose of the mother's flora via the birth canal, setting up the child with a blueprint of microbes that will continue to develop as he or she grows. We pick up additional microbes along the way from our environment, to complete our own individual gut microbiome.

DID YOU KNOW?

Interestingly, where we live in the world shapes the makeup of our gut bacteria. For example, research published in the journal *Nature* in 2012 showed that people living in rural West Africa had a greater diversity of gut bacteria, and also a higher amount of fiber-loving bacteria, than many others in more developed areas. Compare this with First World guts, which showed much less variety, and a dominance of carbohydrate- and protein-loving bacteria. This is indicative of the way that we generally eat in the First World: lots of meat and lots of carbohydrates. Our gut bacteria tend to show that they can adapt to the specific environment and food supply they are given. One solution to our Western lack of gut bacteria diversity proposed by several Stanford University scientists is to consume fermented foods (and drinks).

Gut bacteria, or gut microbiota, are constantly present in our digestive tract, existing happily in a symbiotic relationship with our body. As much as this may sound like a big microbial love-in, it is actually a highly organized and strictly controlled environment. If it starts to suffer, then food intolerances, malnutrition, and disease rear their heads. The concept of being overfed and undernourished is so relevant in modern society. There is an abundance of food; however, what we choose to eat often has the least nutrients. The quality of our food affects our gut bacteria by either nourishing it or degrading it, while at the same time the quality of our gut bacteria has an impact on the level of nutrients able to be absorbed from our food.

It can be quite a delicate balance. Ideally, the friendly bacteria outnumber the unfriendly bacteria, and everyone gets along beautifully. The problem arises when the number of unfriendly bacteria tips the scales in their direction.

Gut bacteria can be divided into three groups:

- Essential or beneficial. Taking up the lion's share of space in a healthy person, beneficial flora are essential to our health and contain the well-known celebrities of the bacteria world, Bifidobacteria and Lactobacillus, but also include Propionibacteria and healthy strains of *E. coli*, Streptococcus, and Enterococcus.

- Opportunistic. The bacteria in this category are kept under tight control in a healthy person, but they can cause disease if allowed to run wild. The culprits include bacteriods, Staphylococcus, Streptococcus, Clostridia, and yeasts, just to name a few. There are about 500 species that we know about thus far, and the combination that they present in can be quite individual.

- Transitional. When the gut is protected by good bacteria, transitional flora pass through like tourists. However, if the gut is damaged or the balance of bacteria is off, this gives them the chance to cause trouble.

What Do Healthy Gut Bacteria Do?

In return for room and board, our gut bacteria work hard! First, they form a coat along the entire intestinal tract. This layer acts as a protective barrier, a security bouncer if you will, between our enterocytes (gut cells) and the food that we eat. If this community of bacteria is not healthy, the gut wall can become malnourished, as it relies on bacteria for up to 70 percent of its nourishment, according to Dr. Natasha McBride in her book *Gut and Psychology Syndrome*. The digestive wall becomes damaged over time, and food is not digested properly. The gut loses its integrity and becomes like my first attempt at knitting—loose and ridden with holes, allowing partially digested proteins and particles into the bloodstream. The immune system in the blood doesn't recognize these partially digested proteins as food, but rather considers them as foreign invaders and mounts an attack against them. From here, low-grade inflammation begins to seep throughout the body, and this may lead to a number of chronic diseases or metabolic syndrome. If the bacteria lining is healthy, it is beautifully and smoothly knitted together and is able to completely digest and absorb the required nutrients—and keep out harmful particles.

On top of this, gut bacteria also produce short-chain fatty acids, which the body can use as fuel to regulate cholesterol metabolism, for hormone production, and to regulate a process called apoptosis, which is programmed cell death. In this way, it can encourage correct development of gut cells and help prevent polyps or diseases like cancer. The production and by-products of these acids also help maintain a healthy gut by keeping the gut acidic. In contrast to the rest of the body, an acidic environment in the gut is a good thing, because it makes an uncomfortable breeding ground for bad bacteria, therefore limiting their growth and activity.

Dr. McBride reports that our gut bacteria also produce antibiotic-like substances that have antifungal and antiviral characteristics. She states that gut bacteria also have the ability to neutralize toxins produced by pathogenic bacteria and

The Lowdown on Gut Cells

Our gut cells, called enterocytes, are extremely specialized and extremely hard-working. They have such a workload, in fact, that they only live for two to three days. At that point, they are so worn out that they are given their gold watch and are shed off by the body. They are replaced by shiny new enterocytes, and the process continues. The cells are continually replaced every couple of days. In order for this process to run smoothly, enterocytes need to have the correct nutrition to reproduce, such as good fats and other vitamins. They also need a healthy gut made up of healthy gut microbes.

Regular consumption of cultured beverages contributes directly to maintaining quality gut health. Numerous animal studies have shown that if the digestive tract is "sterilized" and all bacteria are removed, this entire cycle goes bananas. Cell renewal is interrupted, takes longer, and becomes abnormal, leading cells to become diseased and cancerous. Even though these studies were performed on animals, we can extrapolate that gut bacteria is also absolutely vital for human health.

to synthesize vitamin K_2, amino acids, and B vitamins, including B_1, B_2, B_3, B_5, B_6, folate, and B_{12}. Why is this important? Vitamins, in particular B vitamins, have a short life span in the body. Whether we get these via food or supplementation, there will be times when the body is low in these nutrients. The bacteria enable a steady stream of vitamins, but also allow proper absorption—as long as they are healthy. Without healthy gut bacteria, there is no guarantee that vitamins and minerals will be absorbed, and thus deficiencies can occur.

Iron is one mineral that is particularly compromised by an overgrowth of unhealthy bad bacteria in the gut. The main reason is that the pathogenic bacteria love iron and will consume it all themselves before you even get a look at it. Because of this, iron supplementation will often be literally feeding the pathogenic bacteria and not correcting the problem. If you are low in iron or anemic, it is even more important to correct the balance of microbes in the gut.

How Do You Know If Your Gut Bacteria Are Out of Balance?

Unfortunately, there are many things that can turn this symbiotic relationship sour. Antibiotic use, birth control pills, alcohol, drugs, certain medications, coffee, poor diet, and stress can all play their role in harming our healthy gut flora. Symptoms such as bloating, gas, abdominal discomfort, indigestion, constipation, diarrhea, and vaginal itching or discharge, as well as conditions like irritable bowel syndrome, leaky gut, food intolerances, celiac disease, and presence of Candida (yeast), can all be signs that the scales have tipped in the wrong direction.

Justin Sonnenburg, a Stanford University microbiologist, suggests that a lack of fiber and a diet rich in processed foods and additives are damaging our gut microbiota. In an article in *Nature* in 2012, he also described how the consumption of sterile, mass-produced, calorie-dense foods are making it difficult for our gut bacteria to adapt, and that various species are becoming harder to find as the biodiversity in our guts declines. This means that as most of the food that we eat is sterile, or without good bacteria, we are losing the beautiful array of different species of gut bacteria and along the way altering our very biology. Including cultured beverages as a regular feature in our diet helps to encourage a colorful biodiversity of bacteria within our guts.

Cultured Beverages for Gut Health: An Ecosystem of Love!

Cultured beverages, along with other fermented foods, are a fabulous way to create optimal balance in the gut. It is important to incorporate fermented foods and drinks into our diets frequently, as much of the bacteria in our gut is transient, meaning that it comes in, does its job, and moves on. Daily doses are best to establish fabulous flora.

How Cultured Beverages Assist Digestion

In addition to contributing to the creation of a healthy gut ecosystem, cultured beverages have specific actions that directly help digestive function. First, fermented beverages, via their slightly sour taste, help stimulate saliva and digestive secretions.

Sourness and bitterness are not typically tastes sought after by the general population. We are much more drawn to the sweet and the salty. However, these sour and bitter flavors have a long tradition in digestive health. It is still part of the cultural tradition in many countries, particularly in Europe, to have an aperitif before eating or a digestif after meals, such as vermouth or an herbal liqueur. These are alcoholic beverages traditionally used to enhance appetite and improve digestion.

It is important to note also that all fermented and cultured beverages contain varying amounts of alcohol. The percentage, however, is quite low, at around 0.5 percent, which falls within the range of being labeled a nonalcoholic beverage. There is potential for this percentage to creep higher when fermenting with straight fruit juice, or with the honey mead recipes on pages 170 to 172, which are fermented for much longer periods of time.

In traditional Chinese medicine, sour and bitter flavors are recognized as essential parts of the palate. Bitters are cooling in nature and therefore help reduce inflammation in the body. Paul Pitchford, in his book *Healing with Whole Foods*, talks about bitters being beneficial for bowel function, liver function, and conditions of stagnancy such as constipation.

It is well documented by both traditional and modern herbalists that bitter herbs and flavors increase digestive secretions. The bitter taste receptors on the tongue recognize the bitter flavor and set off a chain reaction that travels along the nerve and hormonal pathways, ending in the stimulation of digestive secretions like stomach acid and pancreatic enzymes.

Fermented beverages play their part here beautifully. One study in the journal *Gut* in 1997 showed that fermented beverages stimulate gastric acid output, along with the release of gastrin, a hormone that stimulates the release of gastric acid from the stomach. Gastrin is also involved in the production of bile by the liver and in the production of some pancreatic enzymes to assist digestion. This happens via the stimulation of the bitter taste receptors, which travel via nerve pathways to stimulate our digestive secretions. Another study in 1999 from the *Journal of Clinical Investigation* showed that it was specifically the maleic acid and succinic acid in fermented beverages that stimulated the gastric acid.

Traditionally, probiotics and cultured beverages have been used to help with the management of common digestive complaints, such as irritable bowel syndrome (IBS), constipation, diarrhea, lactose intolerance, intestinal hyperpermeability (also known as leaky gut syndrome, or the degradation of the gut wall that allows particles through to the bloodstream that should not be able to pass through in a healthy gut), Candida, dysbiosis (an imbalance of bad versus good bacteria in the gut), and gastrointestinal infection.

A French study in *Neurogastroenterology and Motility* in 2012 showed that fermented milk beverages inhibited abdominal pain and protected the gut barrier function in constipated IBS patients. Another study in *Alimentary Pharmacology and Therapeutics* in 2009 recorded improvements in bloating and distension in patients with IBS who used fermented milk beverages.

Kefir: The Champagne of Milks

The first cultured beverage that I will introduce to you is kefir. Kefir is made from small, gelatinous globs called grains. They look a bit like tiny, slimy cauliflower florets, clumped together waiting for a cheese sauce. Sounds appetizing, doesn't it? But like everything, it's what's inside that counts. Mingled among the clumpy grains are a plethora of beneficial bacteria and yeasts. They are self-reproducing, and given the right conditions will continue to do so indefinitely. Kefir involves a community of about thirty different types of microbes that live together in a symbiotic relationship, growing in number with each batch made. The various Lactobacillis species of bacteria are the most prevalent species of bacteria present in kefir, accompanied by beneficial Streptococcus strains, some Lauconostoc species, a number of beneficial yeasts, and also Acetobacter species. A study from the *International Journal of Food Microbiology* in 2006 listed other products formed

Improving Lactose Tolerance

Fermented milk beverages like kefir can also improve lactose intolerance. Gut bacteria, and in particular a healthy strain of *E. coli*, help digest lactose. We normally associate *E. coli* with food-poisoning episodes, but there are a number of strains of *E. coli* that live happily in a healthy gut. Furthermore, these *E. coli* bacteria produce vitamin K_2 and can prevent other pathogenic bacteria from setting up shop in the gut. Dr. Natasha McBride explains that as children, our guts are loaded with beneficial strains of *E. coli* that flourish until antibiotics or other toxins destroy them. Fermenting the milk beverage reduces the lactose, as the bacteria use it up to feed themselves. Research from the *Journal of the American Dietetic Association* published in 2003 shows kefir to improve lactose tolerance.

Fermented beverages both protect and nourish intestinal cells. One study in the *Biological and Pharmacological Bulletin* in 2013 showed kefir in particular to have a protective effect against radiation therapy. The research showed that kefir protects the intestine and promotes the regeneration of the cells. This is fantastic news, and perhaps further research will lead to the more widespread promotion of this information by health professionals for those undergoing radiation treatment.

during the fermentation process, including lactic acid, acetic acid, and pyruvic acid, along with a number of other acids.

Magically, the kefir culture changes liquids such as milk and water into truly powerful health-giving beverages. Once the grains are added to the milk, the hungry beasts begin to consume the sugar (lactose) in the milk. They will continue to feed from the lactose until it is gone. This feeding process produces by-products such as lactic acid, which have their own résumé of goodness we will hear about later.

The end result leaves you with something similar to a drinking yogurt, but a little tarter and with much more bacteria and goodness.

Health Benefits of Kefir

When we consume kefir, it coats the digestive tract in a thin layer of mucus. Normally mucus is not considered a beneficial part of digestion, but in this case, the mucus lays down a bed for the friendly bacteria to settle and colonize. Donna Gates in *The Body Ecology Diet* explains that if we are ingesting other forms of probiotics (such as cultured beverages), this mucus gives them more of an opportunity to establish themselves in our digestive tract. Another study in the *Annals of Nutrition and Metabolism* in 2012 showed the ability of one strain of kefir bacteria in particular, *L. plantaarum*, to have the ability to adhere to the gut wall and protect against pathogenic bacteria.

But the benefits of kefir don't stop there. Kefir is both a prebiotic and a probiotic. A prebiotic is a nondigestible carbohydrate that feeds and nourishes the bacteria and encourages their growth. Other foods that contain prebiotics include raw chicory root, Jerusalem artichoke, raw garlic, raw leeks, raw and cooked onion, dandelion greens, and banana. Fermented dairy products like kefir are a combination of prebiotics and probiotics working together in the same substance, and therefore fall into the category of synbiotics. These items contain the bacteria plus the sustenance that they need to survive.

Kefir contains calcium, potassium, phosphorus, magnesium, zinc, manganese, and molybdenum. The fermentation process of kefir leaves us with B vitamins such as B_{12}, folate, biotin, and B_6. Because kefir is so rich in vitamins and minerals, it assists digestion by providing the essential nutrients needed for the production of digestive juices. Such nutrients are also invaluable in hundreds of other reactions and processes in the body.

For bacteria to do their job, they need to be able to make it through the assault of stomach acid, bile salts, and enzymes thrown at them on their journey through the digestive tract. Some are stronger than others in this capacity. Kefir has a wonderful quality of buffering the bacteria against these elements. In a study in the journal of *Food Microbiology* in 2009, kefir showed an extra protective effect on lactic acid bacteria, allowing them to tolerate higher levels of acidity and also encouraging better adhesion to the gut lining. In this way, kefir functions like a suit of armor, a Velcro suit of armor, both protecting and adhering at the same time.

Another fantastic health benefit of kefir is its antibacterial effect. Several research studies report kefir to exhibit an antibacterial effect on *Listeria monocytogenes* (*Journal of Applied Microbiology*, 2003), *Listeria innocua* (*Journal of Applied Microbiology*, 2000), *Salmonella enteritidis* (*International Journal of Food Microbiology*, 2007), *Staphylococcus areus, Bacillus cereus, E. coli* (*Turkish Microbiological Society*, 2007), and *Candida albicans* (*Brazilian Journal of Microbiology*, 2009). This antibacterial effect from the organic acids produced in the fermentation process works toward preventing gastrointestinal disorders and vaginal infections.

How to Make Kefir

Traditionally, kefir is made using kefir grains to culture a beverage, but there are also starter cultures available for making kefir. The starter culture is a powder made in a laboratory, and it has much fewer strains of bacteria (about eight) than traditional kefir. Another downside of the powdered starter culture is that there are few, if any, yeasts present, and since we don't know the full spectrum of bacteria living in the kefir community, there is in fact no way to make a true powdered form of it. However, this starter culture does make it easy for those who just want to make the odd batch now and then, and it can also culture nondairy varieties of milk more easily.

So take your pick. For the purpose of this book, we'll be looking only at kefir grains.

It may be useful to note that the kefir grains do not contain any actual grain, so they are gluten-free. Kefir can be used to culture a number of different liquids, but it is traditionally used with cow's milk. I recommend using organic milk for culturing kefir. An important point to note is that long-life or ultra-pasteurized (UHT) milk is not recommended for fermenting, as the process that the milk goes through leaves the milk "sterile" and not as amenable to the culture. So read your milk labels to make sure you are not buying ultra-pasteurized milk.

In addition to cow's milk, other milks that can be used to make kefir are goat's milk, sheep's milk, raw milk, and coconut milk. If using nondairy milk, however, it is best to return your grains to a dairy milk every few batches for the best results.

Basic Milk Kefir

This recipe is wonderfully simple. Get this down pat and you are good to go and experiment as you please with other recipes. Drink it on its own or add to smoothies, dressings, and desserts.

1 cup (235 ml) milk

1½ teaspoons milk kefir grains

Glass jar (no lid required), plus a jar with lid for storage

Small piece of cheesecloth, or a paper towel or coffee filter

Rubber band

Fine-mesh strainer

Pour the milk into the first glass jar, and add the kefir grains. Secure the cheesecloth on top with a rubber band and store at room temperature for 12 to 24 hours. This time is dependent on the temperature in your home and also the level of sourness that you desire. It may take up to 48 hours. Taste it periodically to get a feel for what it tastes like at different stages of fermentation, and stop when you reach a point you are happy with. The longer you leave it, the more sour it will become, and the less sugar your kefir will have as the grains feed off the lactose (milk sugar).

Strain the kefir through the mesh strainer into the second glass jar, seal with a lid, and enjoy as is; at this point it is ready to use in other recipes. Your kefir will keep in the refrigerator for about 1 week. Always check your kefir before consuming it, and refrain from drinking any that smells off or rancid.

Transfer the kefir grains left in the strainer to a new jar to begin a new batch. Your kefir grains may continue to multiply and grow, so don't be surprised if your grains double in size over the course of a month. If they don't, this is okay. If you would like to slow down this process once you have enough, or if you are going on vacation and have no one to look after and feed your kefir grains fresh milk, place the grains in a jar and cover with milk. Seal the jar with a lid and place in the refrigerator. The cold will slow the culturing process, and your kefir grains will keep this way for several weeks. If you require a longer amount of storage time, you can either repeat this process or dehydrate your kefir grains—see the FAQs on page 182 for more details.

You can continue to make batch after batch indefinitely. Something to keep in mind is that over time, your kefir may separate into curds and whey. This happens if you allow your kefir to over-culture a little. If you like, you can give it a shake and then drink it as long as it doesn't smell rancid or off. If not, be aware that you should allow less time for your next batch.

What Is Water Kefir (Tibicos)?

As opposed to milk kefir grains, which can be used to culture milk and coconut milk, water kefir grains, also called tibicos, can be used to culture water, coconut water, or juice. The basic idea is to make a sugar water for the culture to thrive on, as the liquid does not have the lactose that is present in milk.

You can use a number of different sugars, but I recommend rapadura sugar, also called panela, or another whole sugar that still has the molasses intact, such as Sucanat. The minerals in the molasses help keep your kefir happy and healthy. You can also use regular white cane sugar if you can't find these whole sugars (or you may use a mix of sugars); either way, organic is ideal.

In an ideal world, it is best to use pure springwater for all your ferments. The chlorine and fluoride in tap water may be damaging to your kefir grains over time; however, if you are only making small batches, this is less of an issue. Boiling tap water before you use it removes the chlorine from water, but be sure to let it cool completely before proceeding. You can also leave the tap water to sit on the counter in an open container for about 12 hours, which will cause the chlorine to dissipate into the air.

Yield 1 cup (235 ml)

Basic Water Kefir

2 cups (475 ml) water

2 tablespoons (26 g) sugar

2 tablespoons (about 20 g) water kefir grains

EQUIPMENT YOU WILL NEED:

Saucepan

Glass jar (no lid required), plus a jar with lid for storage

Small piece of cheesecloth, or a paper towel or coffee filter

Rubber band

Fine-mesh strainer

Put the water into the saucepan and bring to a boil. Remove from the heat, and add the sugar, stirring to dissolve. Let the mixture cool completely; if you don't, you will risk damaging some of the lovely bugs, as they are heat sensitive.

Transfer the water sugar mixture to the first glass jar and add the kefir grains.

Cover with cheesecloth and secure with a rubber band.

Leave the jar at room temperature for 48 hours. You may see bubbles start to form, and the kefir will usually become cloudy in color and taste less sweet than the mixture you started with.

Strain the kefir through the mesh strainer and transfer the fermented kefir to the lidded glass jar, leaving about 1 inch (2.5 cm) of space at the top. You may choose to drink it plain, just as it is, or to proceed to some of the other recipes in this book. I recommend the latter, as plain tibicos is fairly neutral in flavor.

For the second fermentation in other recipes, you may add any flavorings you like. These may include fresh or dried fruit, herbs, spices, or fruit juice. The recipes that follow will provide you with some inspiration, but you can experiment with your own ideas. Once you have added your desired flavoring, allow your brew to ferment for 1 to 3 days (usually 2 days, but this depends on the temperature of your home). The longer you leave it, the more sour-tasting the result will be. After the second fermentation is complete, pop the kefir into the fridge in an airtight jar, and drink within 1 month.

Transfer the kefir grains from the strainer to a new jar to start a new batch.

Your water kefir grains are a living thing. Every few batches you might like to give the grains an extra nutrient boost by adding ¼ teaspoon blackstrap molasses, a piece of organic dried fruit (figs are great), and a slice of organic lemon (don't squeeze). This gives the grains some multivitamins and minerals to keep them happy and healthy. Using half a sterilized eggshell has a similar effect due to the minerals within the eggshell. To sterilize an eggshell, crack an uncooked egg and save for later use. Place the shell in a small saucepan of boiling water for a few minutes. Then just pop it into the batch while you are fermenting the grains, and remove and discard it at the end.

Makes 2 cups (475 ml)

Basic Coconut Milk Kefir

Using coconut milk creates a delicious, creamy kefir that you can use as a base for smoothies, as a topping for desserts, or even as an addition to your coffee or tea.

1 cup (235 ml) coconut milk, unsweetened, or make your own from a fresh young coconut (see Note)

1½ teaspoons milk kefir grains

EQUIPMENT YOU WILL NEED:

Glass jar (no lid required), plus a jar with lid for storage

Small piece of cheesecloth, or a paper towel or coffee filter

Rubber band

Fine-mesh strainer

Pour the milk into the first glass jar, and add the kefir grains.

Secure the cheesecloth on top with the rubber band and store at room temperature for 12 to 24 hours. This time is dependent on the temperature in your home and also the level of sourness that you desire. It may take up to 48 hours. The kefir will start to thicken after about 12 hours, so check it periodically to get a feel for what it tastes like at different stages of fermentation, and stop when you reach a consistency and taste you are happy with.

Strain the kefir through the mesh strainer into the lidded glass jar, and keep in the refrigerator for about 1 week.

Transfer the kefir grains to a new jar to begin a new batch.

Note: You can also make coconut milk kefir using a whole fresh young coconut. Just open the coconut and pour the water inside into a blender. Scoop out the white flesh from inside the coconut and add that to the blender too. Blend until smooth. Now use 1 cup (235 ml) of this liquid in the recipe.

Although this recipe uses coconut milk, it still uses tibicos that have been "raised" on milk. If you require a truly dairy-free option, the website culturesforhealth.com has the wonderful suggestion of mixing ¼ cup (60 ml) finished fermented water kefir (not the grains) with 2 to 4 cups (475 to 946 ml) coconut milk, and then allowing it to ferment for 24 hours.

Yield: 1 cup (235 ml)

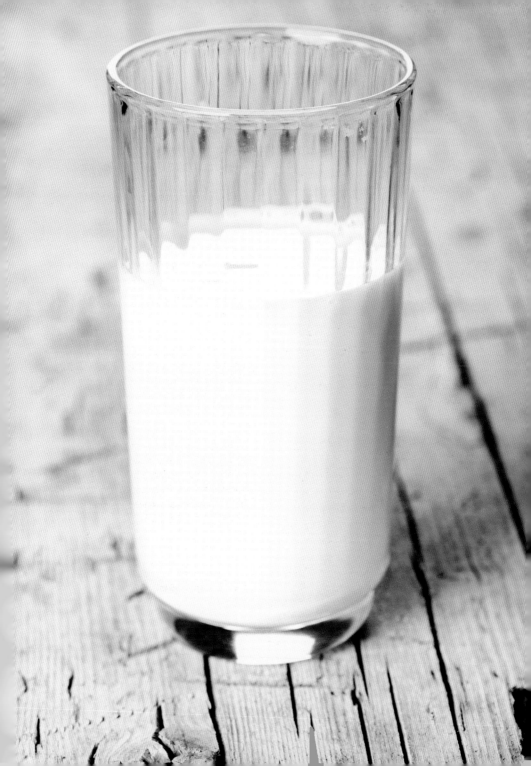

Basic Coconut Water Kefir

4 cups (946 ml) coconut water

2 tablespoons (about 20 g) water kefir grains

EQUIPMENT YOU WILL NEED:

Glass jar (no lid required), plus a jar with lid for storage

Small piece of cheesecloth, or a paper towel or coffee filter

Rubber band

Fine-mesh strainer

Add the coconut water and water kefir grains to the first glass jar, cover with cheesecloth and seal with the rubber band, and leave to ferment at room temperature for 24 to 48 hours.

Strain the kefir grains through the mesh strainer and transfer the fermented kefir to the lidded glass jar, leaving about 1 inch (2.5 cm) of space at the top. Add any flavorings you like (fruit, herbs, juice) and allow to ferment for 1 to 3 days (usually 2 days, but this depends on the temperature of your home).

After fermentation is complete, keep in the refrigerator for up to 1 month.

Transfer the kefir grains to a new jar to start a new batch.

Yield: 4 cups (946 ml)

Introducing Kombucha

Kombucha is an ancient, sour, and slightly sweet elixir originating in Asia and brewed using a living, somewhat crazy-looking spongy disk. The disk, or pacake-shaped agent, used to ferment kombucha is referred to as a "mother" or SCOBY (Symbiotic Colony of Bacteria and Yeast).

Traditionally made from black tea and sugar, the SCOBY ferments the tea but also reproduces itself, forming another mother. It may sound like something out of an alien movie, and there is often a bit of jaw-dropping action when you see it for the first time, but this phenomenon is such a winner that you will forgive its weirdness. So, after completing the fermenting process, you end up with two mothers and a slightly sweet, slightly sour elixir that is a nutritional and gut-healing powerhouse!

As with kefir, it is best to use organic sugar, either rapadura sugar or white cane sugar, to make kombucha. Artificial sweeteners will not work. Honey is controversial. The issue is that honey is naturally antibacterial and contains bacteria that may compete with that in the SCOBY. I have used honey successfully, but I never do more than one batch with honey at a time, in order to preserve the SCOBY.

It's also best, again as with kefir, to use pure springwater. If you use tap water and boil it to remove the chlorine, be sure to let it cool completely before adding your SCOBY.

Black tea is the best tea to use for kombucha brewing, but green tea, white tea, and rooibos also work, as well as yerba maté. Pu-erh tea is a fermented Chinese variety of tea that is often recommended for making kombucha. In pu-erh tea, the natural microbes living on the tea ferment the leaves. For more about which teas work for making kombucha, see the FAQs on page 178.

Basic Kombucha

If this is the first time you are making kombucha and you don't have any tea left over from a previous batch, use the liquid that came with your SCOBY when you received it.

4 cups (946 ml) water

¼ cup (50 g) organic sugar

2 organic black tea bags

1 kombucha SCOBY

½ cup (120 ml) kombucha tea from a previous batch

EQUIPMENT YOU WILL NEED:

Saucepan

Wide-mouth glass jar (no lid required), plus a jar with lid for storage

Clean kitchen towel

Place the water in the saucepan and bring to a boil. Turn off the heat. Add the sugar, stirring until dissolved.

Place the tea bags into the saucepan and leave to brew until the tea cools to room temperature.

Once cool, remove the tea bags and transfer the tea to the wide-mouth glass jar.

Add the SCOBY and the kombucha tea from the previous batch.

Cover with the clean kitchen towel or an unbleached coffee filter or paper towel, and place in a warm spot away from sunlight (ideally 70° to 85°F, or 21° to 29°C). The top of the refrigerator is a great spot!

The time it takes your kombucha to ferment will vary slightly depending on the temperature; the warmer the temperature, the faster the process. Also, the longer you leave it, the more sour your tea will become, as the bacteria are consuming the sugar. Be aware that the SCOBY can move around in the jar. It may sit at the bottom, float in the middle, or hang out on top and fuse to the second developing SCOBY. All of this is fine. The end result should be slightly sour and a little fizzy.

After 5 to 7 days, you will notice the beginnings of the new mother forming on the top of the liquid. You can start tasting your brew at this point with a straw, so as not to disturb your developing SCOBY. Don't poke at it; the more you move it, the more likely it is to break apart, and the longer it will take to develop into a pretty new mother.

You may choose to leave your kombucha for up to 14 days or longer, depending on the ambient temperature and how sour you like it. Once it is ready, with clean hands, carefully take out the mother and baby SCOBY, set aside ½ cup (120 ml) of the mixture to culture your next brew, and transfer the finished kombucha into the lidded glass jar. Store in the refrigerator for up to 1 month.

To make a new batch, you can use the original mother or the new mother. Each time you culture, you will grow a new SCOBY, and your original will grow another layer and thicken slightly. How amazing is that?

Second Fermentation

As with your kefir, you can put your finished kombucha through a second ferment, which is where you can get creative and fancy with different flavorings.

Simply decant your kombucha into a jar with a lid. Add your flavorings, pop the lid on tightly, and allow to ferment at room temperature for another 1 to 2 days. This process will also allow your kombucha to become fizzy, as the bacteria and yeasts feed on the flavorings that you have added. Be sure to check on your ferment, as you will need to burp your bottle from time to time to make sure you don't acquire exploding kombucha wallpaper. To do this, simply open the jar and let a little air out. Just like burping a baby, really! Once your second fermentation is complete, you can store your kombucha in the refrigerator, and this will slow down the fermentation process.

How to Look After Your SCOBY

You can reuse the same SCOBY for years. Here are some hot tips to keep your SCOBY beautiful:

- Always use clean hands when handling it. If you notice black or green patches, you have contamination, and you will need to throw it away and get a new mother.

- Don't wash or rinse your SCOBY between uses.

- Always use glass jars for storage. The acids in the kombucha will leach out chemicals from plastic.

- If you want to slow down your culturing factory, pop your SCOBY along with some kombucha into an airtight glass jar in the refrigerator. The cold temperature will slow down the fermentation process. You can leave your SCOBY here safely for a long time if needed. Some have reported not using their SCOBY for years, and then using it again with no problem.

- You may use honey in place of the sugar if you prefer, but because it has antibacterial properties, it has the potential to compete with and damage your growing friendly bacteria. Make sure you always have another SCOBY that has only been fed sugar as a backup.

Yield: About 4¼ cups (1 liter)

Putting It into Practice

- A healthy gut is essential to the health of our whole body. If our digestive system is not in balance, we may develop digestive symptoms or disease throughout the body. Healthy gut bacteria is absolutely essential for good gut health.

- Gut bacteria protect, feed, and nourish the gut lining and aid in the digestion, absorption, and processing of nutrients. They produce enzymes, acids, and other by-products that help regulate hormone production, cholesterol metabolism, correct cell function, vitamin synthesis, and the neutralizing of toxins. Gut bacteria also play a large role in the immune system, detoxification, healthy skin, and a healthy mind.

- Symptoms of an overgrowth of unhealthy gut bacteria may include bloating, gas, abdominal discomfort, indigestion, irritable bowel syndrome, Candida (yeast), and food intolerances.

- Fermented beverages assist in the creation of a healthy gut ecosystem and therefore may help with all of the above issues. They protect and nourish the gut, stimulate digestive secretions, improve liver function, and can reduce lactose intolerance.

 DID YOU KNOW?

There are currently some exciting new areas of research being explored whereby good bacteria can assist in other, less traditional, applications. These include mastitis, endometriosis, prevention of diabetes and gestational diabetes, prevention of postpartum obesity, and management of anxiety disorders and depression.

Jason Hawrelak, who has his PhD in intestinal dysbiosis and the clinical applications of prebiotics and probiotics, states that there are four essential traits that probiotics should have. These are the ability to adhere to the gut mucosa, stabilize gastric acid, colonize the intestinal tract, and show clinically documented health effects. Fermented beverages tick all of these boxes—and more!

Cultured and Fermented Beverage Recipes for Healthy Digestion

Chai Kefir

Chai is an Indian spiced tea that has really increased in popularity in the past few years. And rightly so, because it's delicious! Full of warming spices to aid digestion, it is traditionally brewed in milk and served warm. To preserve the lovely bacteria in our kefir, this is a cold version. The spice mix will keep in an airtight jar for months. Feel free to use it to make traditional chai by adding ¼ to ½ teaspoon per cup of milk (any kind) and gently bringing almost to a boil in a small saucepan before adding black tea.

2 cups (475 ml) Basic Milk Kefir (page 24) or Basic Coconut Milk Kefir (page 28)

½ to 1 teaspoon Chai Spice Blend (recipe follows) or 2 chai tea bags

Pour the kefir into a jar, add the chai spices or tea bags, cover loosely with cheesecloth or the lid (but not airtight), and allow to sit at room temperature for 12 to 24 hours. Stop the process once you reach the desired tartness.

Strain the mixture to remove the spices, or remove the tea bags, and keep the chai kefir in the refrigerator for up to 5 days.

Yield: 2 cups (475 ml)

Chai Spice Blend

1 cinnamon stick

5 whole cloves

6 cardamom pods

4 black peppercorns

1 teaspoon ground ginger

1 teaspoon fennel seeds

Grind the spices in a mortar and pestle or a spice grinder. Store in an airtight container.

Makes about 1½ tablespoons (about 10 g)

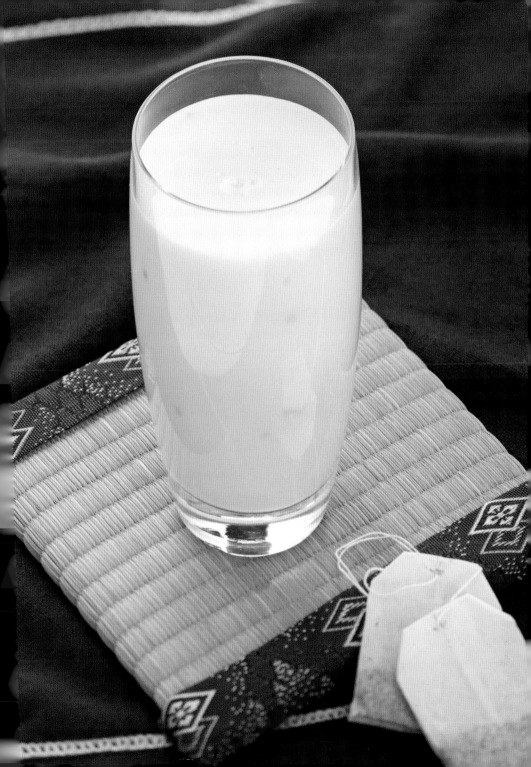

Apple Pie Kefir with Crunchy Granola Topping

There is something about apple pie that is universally comforting and homey. In the warmer months, I like to change up the ingredients in this pie-inspired drink a bit and use water kefir or coconut water kefir instead of the milk. The topping on this one makes it just that little bit closer to the real thing!

2 tablespoons (10 g) rolled oats

2 tablespoons (10 g) unsweetened coconut flakes

2 tablespoons (14 g) coarsely chopped raw unsalted almonds

1 cup (235 ml) Basic Milk Kefir (page 24) or Basic Coconut Milk Kefir (page 28)

1 apple, cored and coarsely chopped (preferably organic)

½ teaspoon ground cinnamon

¼ teaspoon ground nutmeg

¼ teaspoon pure vanilla extract

1 tablespoon (15 ml) pure maple syrup (optional)

Preheat the oven to 350°F (180°C, or gas mark 4). Place the oats, coconut flakes, and almonds on a baking sheet and bake for 12 minutes, or until the coconut is just starting to brown a little. Remove from the oven and allow to cool.

Add the kefir, apple, cinnamon, nutmeg, vanilla, and maple syrup to a blender and blend until smooth.

Pour into a glass, top with the topping mix, and enjoy!

Yield: 1½ cups (355 ml)

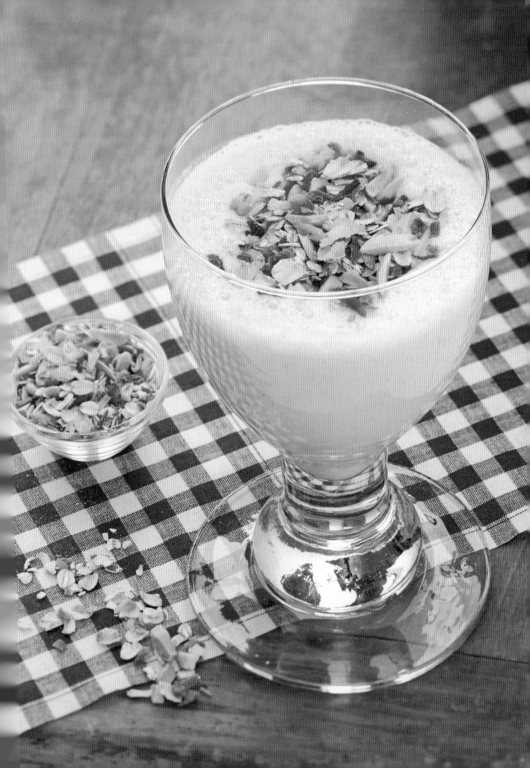

Iced Cacao Kefir Frappé

Refreshing, nourishing, and delicious, this is a great drink to make in the afternoon to replace that second coffee that might be tempting you. Especially in the warmer months, its frappé-type consistency is a fun and enticing way to get your good bacteria!

2 cups (475 ml) Basic Milk Kefir (page 24)

About 20 ice cubes

¼ cup (24 g) raw cacao powder

2 to 3 tablespoons (30 to 45 ml) pure maple syrup

1 teaspoon pure vanilla extract or vanilla powder/paste

Place all of the ingredients in a blender and blend on high speed until smooth. You may want to do this in smaller batches to preserve the blades of your blender. Enjoy right away.

Yield: 3½ cups (825 ml)

Cayenne Lemon Kombucha

The ultimate metabolism party starter, this drink combines cayenne and lemon, a zingy combination to energize your day.

2 cups (475 ml) Basic Kombucha (page 32)

Zest of ½ lemon (preferably organic)

¼ teaspoon cayenne pepper

Place all of the ingredients into a clean glass jar, leaving at least 1 inch (2.5 cm) of space at the top. Put the lid on and keep at room temperature and out of direct sunlight for 1 to 3 days.

Once this second fermentation is complete, strain out the lemon zest and transfer your kombucha to an airtight bottle. Store in the refrigerator for up to 1 month.

Yield: 2 cups (475 ml)

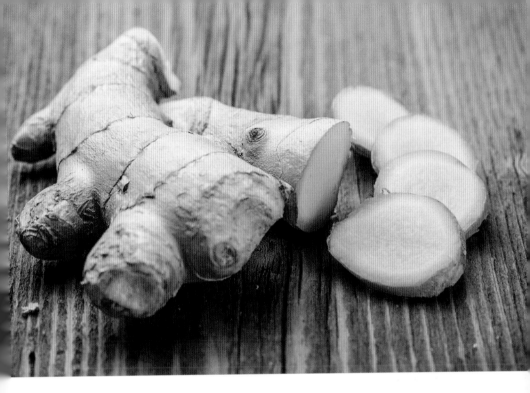

Ginger Kombucha

Straight up ginger! This makes a powerful digestive aid. Anti-inflammatory and antispasmodic, ginger brings a warming energy to the gut, and it can also aid with nausea.

2 cups (475 ml) Basic Kombucha (page 32)

6 to 8 slices fresh ginger (do not peel)

Place both ingredients into a clean glass jar, leaving at least 1 inch (2.5 cm) of space at the top. Put the lid on and keep at room temperature and out of direct sunlight for 1 to 3 days.

Once this second fermentation is complete, strain out the ginger and transfer your kombucha to an airtight bottle. Store in the refrigerator for up to 1 month.

Yield: 2 cups (475 ml)

Spiced Pear Cider Kombucha

If autumn were a drink, this would be it: seasonal pears with lovely rich spices. This recipe makes me want to put my slippers on and curl up under a blanket on the couch.

2 cups (475 ml) Basic Kombucha (page 32)

½ organic pear, coarsely chopped (preferably organic)

1 (1-inch, or 2.5-cm) piece cinnamon stick

3 whole cloves

⅛ teaspoon allspice (optional)

Place all of the ingredients into a clean glass jar, leaving at least 1 inch (2.5 cm) of space at the top. Put the lid on and keep at room temperature and out of direct sunlight for 1 to 3 days.

Once this second fermentation is complete, strain out the fruit and spices and transfer your kombucha to an airtight bottle. Store in the refrigerator for up to 1 month.

Yield: 2 cups (475 ml)

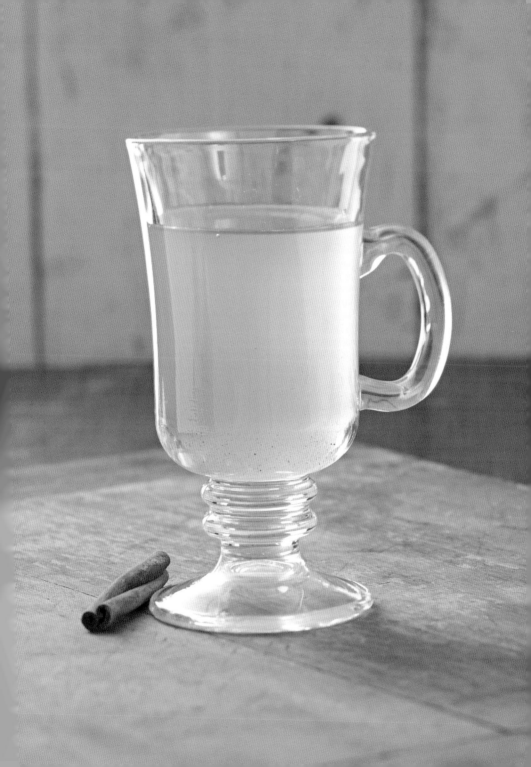

Rose Water Kefir

This is such a pretty drink. I am a sucker for rose water. It has a lovely floral flavor that you need to be careful not to overdo, or you will end up with something like potpourri. Rose water is beautiful with chocolate, and sometimes I like to add a couple of teaspoons of cacao nibs to this infusion for fun.

1 cup (235 ml) Basic Water Kefir (page 26)

7 or 8 drops rose water

4 dried rosebuds from a tea or other food-safe source (optional, but gorgeous)

2 teaspoons cacao nibs (optional)

Place all of the ingredients into a glass jar, leaving 1 inch (2.5 cm) of space at the top, and put the lid on. Keep the jar at room temperature and out of direct sunlight for 2 days.

Strain out the rosebuds, or add them to the serving glass as a garnish. Enjoy right away or store in an airtight bottle in the refrigerator for up to 1 month.

Yield: 1 cup (235 ml)

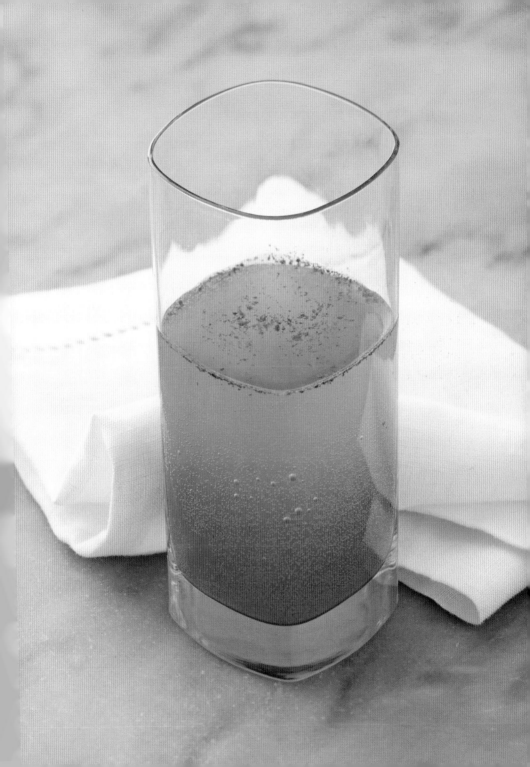

Blueberry Basil Kefir

A wonderful flavor combination makes this drink refreshing and delicious.

1 cup (235 ml) Basic Water Kefir (page 26) or Basic Coconut Water Kefir (page 30)

2 tablespoons (18 g) blueberries (preferably organic)

12 small fresh basil leaves

Place all of the ingredients into a glass jar, leaving 1 inch (2.5 cm) of space at the top, and put the lid on. Keep the jar at room temperature and out of direct sunlight for 2 days.

Strain out the blueberries and basil and enjoy right away or store in an airtight bottle in the refrigerator for up to 1 month.

Yield: 1 cup (235 ml)

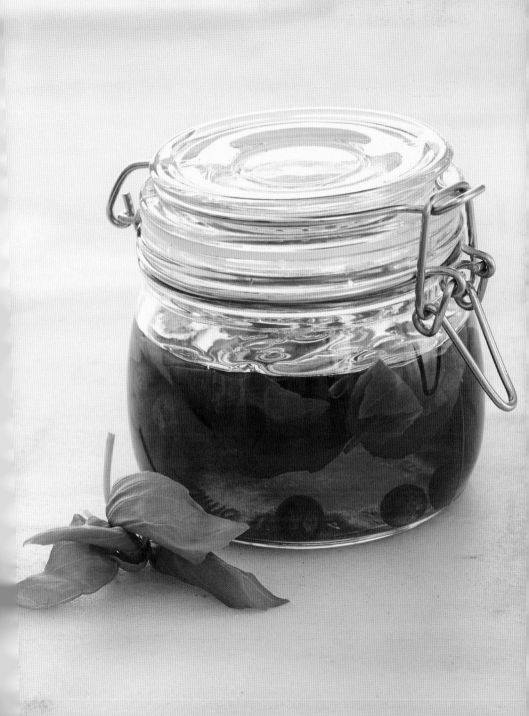

Cinnamon Plum Kombucha

Cinnamon and plum are a wonderful combination, and with the added sourness of kombucha, I think this drink is a winner.

2 cups (475 ml) Basic Kombucha (page 32)

3 or 4 plums, coarsely chopped (preferably organic)

1 (2-inch, or 5-cm) piece cinnamon stick

Place all of the ingredients into a clean glass jar, leaving at least 1 inch (2.5 cm) of space at the top. Put the lid on and keep at room temperature and out of direct sunlight for 1 to 3 days.

Once this second fermentation is complete, strain out the fruit and cinnamon and transfer your kombucha to an airtight bottle. Store in the refrigerator for up to 1 month.

Yield: 2 cups (475 ml)

Fig Vanilla Kombucha

This recipe uses organic dried figs, which contain a surprisingly high amount of calcium. This recipe is also amazing with water kefir or coconut water kefir—it tastes like creamy soda. Just replace the kombucha with the same amount of kefir.

2 cups (475 ml) Basic Kombucha (page 32)

2 figs (preferably organic)

½ vanilla bean, split

Place all of the ingredients into a clean glass jar, leaving at least 1 inch (2.5 cm) of space at the top. Put the lid on and keep at room temperature and out of direct sunlight for 1 to 3 days.

Once this second fermentation is complete, strain out the figs and vanilla bean and transfer your kombucha to an airtight bottle. Store in the refrigerator for up to 1 month.

Yield: 2 cups (475 ml)

Rejuvelac

Rejuvelac is a sprouted grain beverage. Although it's generally made with wheat berries, I have used spelt berries for this recipe. You first need to sprout the grain, and then soak it, and then you can drink the water that has gained all the lovely benefits. Sprouting grains allows them to reach their highest nutritional potential and makes them easier to digest. Fermenting them further leaves you with a veritable explosion of goodness, including natural enzymes from the grain, vitamins (especially B vitamins), and, of course, microbial benefits.

1 cup (180 g) spelt berries

Water as needed

To sprout the berries, put the spelt into a 1-liter jar and fill with enough water to cover. Place cheesecloth over the top to keep any bugs out, and leave for 8 to 10 hours or overnight at room temperature.

Drain off the water, then rinse the spelt and drain again. Leave the jar with the spelt berries at a slight angle for 2 days, coming back to rinse and drain again at least twice a day.

Once the spelt has begun to sprout, rinse thoroughly one last time. Fill the jar with water and soak for 48 hours.

You now have your finished rejuvelac. There may be a white foamy layer on the surface of the water; if so, just skim this off carefully with a spoon. Strain the rejuvelac and store in an airtight bottle in the refrigerator for up to 1 month.

Rejuvelac should be slightly sweet, cloudy, and sometimes fizzy, with a grassy, tart but not too sour taste. If it smells cheesy, you have probably left your grain for too long in the sprouting phase and it may have started to mold. If this is the case, you will need to start again with new grain. Any sign of black, green, or blue mold is no good.

Yield: 4¼ cups (1 liter)

CHAPTER 2

Culturing a Healthy Immune System

The immune system is a highly organized, amazingly busy system of tissues, organs, cells, and molecules that work together to protect our body from disease and infection. It controls the way that we respond to foreign substances in the body, including food and airborne substances. It also coordinates our reaction to microbial pathogens that we come into contact with daily, as well as more chronic immune assaults such as cancer.

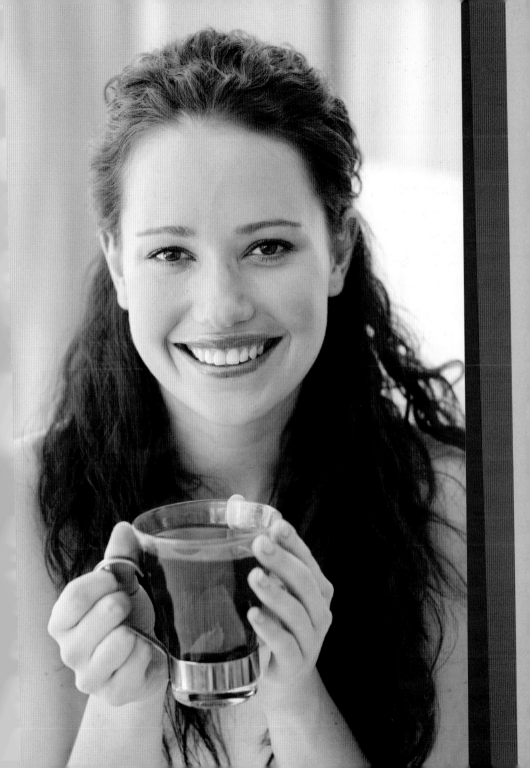

The immune response itself can be split into two main categories: innate/nonspecific immunity and adaptive/acquired immunity.

Innate immunity involves the skin and mucous membranes as our first line of defense. It is our "customs security" to make sure that no shady characters are allowed into the body. This first line of innate defense includes mucus to trap pathogens in its sticky trap, urine to flush out invaders via the kidneys, vomiting to eradicate microbes, and acidic vaginal secretions, which prevent the growth of unwanted bacteria.

If, for some reason, our customs security team is not functioning optimally, is short staffed, hungover, or distracted, a second wave of innate defense comes into play and airport security is initiated. Antimicrobial proteins, natural killer cells, and phagocytes are released to track down pathogens and eliminate them. Inflammation also plays an important role here, setting off a reaction of redness, pain, swelling, and heat to encourage tissue repair.

The second category of immune response is adaptive immunity. Whereas the body mounts a general response in innate immunity, adaptive immunity is extremely precise. This arm of immunity actually remembers the invading pathogen, so that if it invades again, there is a more rapid and virulent defense response than the first time. A photo has been circulated among officials, so to speak, and the team now knows exactly who to look for.

T Helper Cells

There is another layer on top of this. The innate immune response contains cells called antigen presenting cells (APC), whose job it is to identify the pathogen (antigen) and alert the adaptive immune response as to what sort of invader they are dealing with. The adaptive immunity then sends in the T helper cells: Th1 and Th2. Any virus, bacteria, fungi, or cancer cells are Th1's domain, whereas any blood-borne disease is Th2's responsibility. In a healthy immune system, they are balanced, but if imbalance occurs and either one becomes dominant, the body begins attacking itself. Autoimmune disease is a good example of Th1 dominance, whereas asthma, eczema, and food allergies are examples of Th2 dominance.

The lymphatic system is extremely important to immunity, as it coordinates specific immune responses and release of molecules to protect against microbes and abnormal cells. Like a big stage production, this show is made up of a dedicated and hardworking cast involving the lymphatic vessels, thymus gland, lymph nodes and nodules, spleen, bone marrow, and white blood cells.

How Do Gut Bacteria Affect the Immune System?

The bacteria in the gut play a crucial role in this production via their engagement with lymphoid tissue. The main site of mucosal immunity in the gut is called the gut-associated lymphoid tissue (GALT) and produces huge numbers of lymphocytes and immunoglobulins, such as secretory immunoglobulin A (IgA). IgA is the most abundantly produced immunoglobulin in the body and helps protect against microbial invasion of the gut lining and also against pathogenic bacteria. It is found throughout the body in saliva, sweat, tears, the nose, throat, bladder, vagina, and breast milk, but at least 80 percent is located in the GALT. A study in the *American Journal of Clinical Nutrition* in 2004 states that IgA is reliant on good bacteria in the gut for its production, and that without healthy gut bacteria, our ability to produce IgA diminishes dramatically. We need a healthy supply of IgA, as it protects the mucous membranes from harmful bacteria and other pathogens both within our body and from external invaders hitching a ride with our food.

Other immune cells are also affected by a lack of good bacteria in the gut. As reported in the *American Journal of Nutrition* in 2003, without beneficial bacteria, the intestinal immune system is left underdeveloped, and certain cells such as neutrophils and macrophages have a reduced efficacy.

And it's not just in the digestive system that gut bacteria have an influence on immunity. The entire body suffers if the balance of good versus bad bacteria is out of line.

Culturing a Healthy Immune System with Fermented Beverages

Cultured beverages can be of great assistance in keeping our immune system strong. A study in the journal *Immunobiology* in 2006 reported that the by-products produced during the fermentation of beverages have the potential to improve both nonspecific and adaptive immunity in both humans and animals. The study stated that fermented dairy products like kefir can increase the number of IgA cells in the gut mucosa and also the bronchial mucosa. Further, such fermented dairy products can improve the function of immune cells in the lining of the digestive organs and lungs. Research published in the *Journal of Immunology* in 2008 shows the production of higher levels of anti-inflammatory cytokines, or molecules, in response to the lactic acid bacteria from fermented beverages.

Enemies of Our Gut Bacteria

Antibiotics are enemy number one to gut bacteria. Almost everyone has taken a course of them at some time, and we are also exposed to them via our food. Farmed animals given antibiotics pass it on via their meat, milk, and eggs, and some vegetables and grains are sprayed with antibiotics to reduce disease. This can make them difficult to avoid. They can, of course, at times be a necessary and life-saving part of treatment, but the collateral damage is, among other things, the loss of healthy gut bacteria.

Unfortunately, antibiotics are not selective in only killing a certain specific bacterial strain or virus. They often have a blanket approach, taking out a number of strains of good bacteria along the way. When the bacteria are killed off, it leaves a place in the gut lining wide open. This is a crucial time to bring in plenty of healthy bacteria to make sure they are the ones that take up residence. After antibiotic treatment, it can take months for bacteria to recover; an article in the *International Society for Microbial Ecology* in 2007 states that it takes up to two years for some strains to recover. A more recent article in *Nature* in 2011 suggests that some strains of bacteria may never recover.

A study in the journal *Gut* in 2012 showed that after antibiotic treatment, the reduced uptake of iron diminished the capacity to digest certain foods and produce certain molecules. The reduced iron uptake is due to the overgrowth of iron-loving bacteria that can make themselves at home after a course of antibiotics. So taking iron supplements for anemia in these cases would be feeding the unhealthy bacteria rather than just correcting the iron deficiency.

Fermented beverages can help restore gut microflora after antibiotics, and there is also research to show their benefit during a course of antibiotics. A study in the *Journal of Dairy Research* in 2011 showed kefir to shorten the duration of antibiotic-associated diarrhea and to improve gastrointestinal symptoms. An earlier study in

2007 in the *Canadian Journal of Gastroenterology* showed kefir to be safe and effective in the prevention of antibiotic-associated diarrhea, which is mostly caused by a particular bacteria called *Clostridium difficile*. Clostridium species are resistant to antibiotics, and so the best way to deal with them is to overshadow them with good bacteria. One study in *Letters in Applied Biology* in 2002 showed kefir to significantly increase the number of lactic acid bacteria in the mucosa of the gut, and to decrease Clostridia bacteria a hundredfold.

Another article in the *Journal of Medicinal Food* in 2011 showed kefir to improve not only the tolerability but also the effectiveness of antibiotics. Potentially, this may lead to a lower required antibiotic dose, which would be a wonderful step in the right direction. Let's hope that there will be further research in this area. Perhaps the next time we fill a prescription for antibiotics, we can also treat ourselves to a good dose of kefir to improve results.

Allergies, Immunity, and Gut Bacteria: Let Them Eat Dirt!

The prevalence of allergies in developed nations has exploded over the past thirty or so years. The first theory to propose a cause for this was the "Hygiene Hypothesis." Pointing the finger at overenthusiastic use of antibiotics and

 DID YOU KNOW?

It is not only antibiotics that harm our precious internal ecosystem. Painkillers, steroids, oral contraceptive pills, and a number of other drugs all damage gut bacteria. Dr. Natasha McBride claims these cases of dysbiosis, or unbalanced bacteria in the gut, are the most severe and the most resistant to treatment.

Stress also invites itself to the party. A study in the *American Journal of Psychology* in 2006 discovered that stress can actually alter gut wall function, making the wall more permeable and increasing the likelihood of developing food allergies. Another article in 2002 in the journal *Gastroenterology* showed that chronic psychological stress leads to intestinal inflammation and impairs the ability of the gut bacteria to defend themselves against pathogens.

antibacterial cleaning products, this theory ties the limited exposure to pathogens during childhood to the development of a compromised immune system. Bugs that children would typically cross paths with while routinely playing in the dirt or sharing toys with the family cat are now commonly a thing of the past as we rush to sanitize our world. This lack of immune sensitization steers the body toward Th2 dominance. As most allergies result from Th2 dominance, this theory can possibly help explain their increase. The theory gained further credibility in the late 1990s, when researchers in Sweden discovered that typical gut bacteria colonize the guts of infants in Pakistan earlier than they do in Sweden. The study suggested that this delay affects the ability to deal with common, harmless antigens such as pollen and food.

Building on this idea, more demographic information listed in a paper in *Advances in Experimental Medicine and Biology* in 2008 shows children living in cities or built-up areas of Europe with a different profile of microbes in their stools and a far greater incidence of allergies compared with children living in rural areas of Africa.

It is the gut bacteria that regulate the way we respond to an attack on our immune system. If there is an imbalance and the beneficial bacteria are not there to guide the immune cell correctly on how to respond, immune hypersensitivity can occur, and the immune system launches attacks against harmless substances such as pollen or nuts, or against itself.

Given that the healthy human body contains up to ten times more bacteria than cells, it is incredible to think that the immune system largely either ignores or tolerates these microbes. Not only does the immune system need to recognize invading pathogens and deal with them, but it also needs to be able to recognize the resident bacteria as "self." The interaction between the immune system and the microbial cells sets up the way that we respond to external stimuli, and a breakdown in this relationship gives rise to conditions such as autoimmunity.

As Joel Kimmons, epidemiologist and nutrition scientist, says, our gut bacteria are continually reading the environment and responding; they are a microbial mirror of the changing world. Because they evolve so quickly, they assist our bodies in responding to the environment. Gut bacteria are incredible adaptive and versatile, able to swap genes and DNA among themselves and to come up with exactly the right gene required to deal with incoming molecules. An example of this is the ability of the Japanese to be able to extract certain nutrients from seaweed that the rest of the world cannot extract well. A 2010 study in *Nature* tells how the Japanese people have acquired a special type of gut bacteria from marine microbes that carry a gene enabling the breakdown of seaweed—in particular, nori—allowing better use of the nutrients found within.

Putting It into Practice

- The immune system comprises two main categories: innate/nonspecific immunity and adaptive/acquired immunity. Innate immunity is our first line of defense, mounting a general response to any invading pathogens. Adaptive immunity is extremely precise and remembers pathogens so that if they invade a second time, there is a quicker and stronger defense response.

- Gut bacteria play a crucial role in supporting the immune system via their engagement with the gut-associated lymphoid tissue (GALT), which produces huge numbers of lymphocytes and immunoglobulins, helping to protect against microbial invasion of the gut lining and also against pathogenic bacteria.

- Antibiotics, painkillers, oral contraceptive pills, and other over-the-counter drugs all play a role in damaging our gut bacteria, as does stress.

- Gut bacteria regulate the way we respond to an attack on our immune system in the form of allergies. If there is an imbalance and the beneficial bacteria are not there to guide the immune cells correctly on how to respond, the immune system launches attacks against harmless substances such as pollen or nuts, or against itself.

- Fermented beverages help keep our immune system strong by improving both nonspecific and adaptive immunity, improving the function of immune cells, and encouraging the production of higher levels of anti-inflammatory molecules. They also help restore gut microflora after antibiotic use and reduce any associated digestive side effects while taking them.

Cultured and Fermented Beverage Recipes for a Healthy Immune System

Ginger and Goji Berry Kombucha

I love this recipe. Goji berries are so delicious when given the chance to rehydrate, not to mention the swag of nutritional benefits they bring along with them, such as a huge antioxidant profile, protein, vitamin C, and carotenoids. This is the perfect drink to rehydrate with after being out in the sun.

2 cups (475 ml) Basic Kombucha (page 32)

8 to 10 slices fresh ginger (do not peel)

3 to 4 teaspoons (7.5 to 9 g) dried goji berries

Place the kombucha into a clean glass jar, leaving at least 1 inch (2.5 cm) of space at the top. Add the ginger and goji berries and put the lid on.

Keep at room temperature and out of direct sunlight for 1 to 3 days. This will depend on the temperature of your home. Your kombucha will start to carbonate and get a little fizzy as the good bugs start to eat the new sugar from the ginger and goji berries.

Once this second fermentation is complete, strain out the ginger and goji berries and transfer your kombucha to an airtight bottle. Store in the refrigerator for up to 1 month.

Yield: 2 cups (475 ml)

Carrot, Grapefruit, and Ginger Kombucha

This zingy little number is as tasty as it is healthy. If you are using freshly squeezed carrot juice, there may be some separation in the drink, which is normal. Just give it a good stir before drinking.

1 cup (235 ml) Basic Kombucha (page 32)

¼ cup (60 ml) carrot juice

1 teaspoon freshly squeezed grapefruit juice

1 or 2 slices fresh ginger (do not peel)

Place the kombucha into a clean glass jar, leaving at least 1 inch (2.5 cm) of space at the top. Add the carrot juice, grapefruit juice, and ginger, and put the lid on.

Keep at room temperature and out of direct sunlight for 1 to 2 days. This will depend on the temperature of your home.

Once this second fermentation is complete, strain out the ginger and transfer your kombucha to an airtight bottle. Store in the refrigerator for up to 1 month.

Yield: 1¼ cups (285 ml)

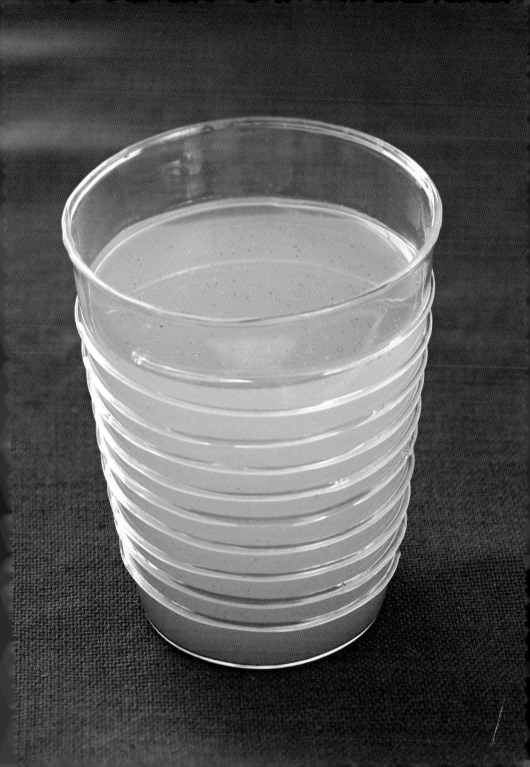

Spirulina Kefir

Spirulina is my favorite green powder. It is an alga, and it happens to be high in protein and contains omega-3, omega-6, and omega-9 fatty acids, as well as a high concentration of iron and nutrients such as B vitamins and vitamins C, D, A, and E. It also has an incredible calcium content and is a fantastic antioxidant. It's no wonder that increased energy is one of the side effects! This recipe also works well with kombucha, if you prefer.

1 cup (235 ml) Basic Coconut Water Kefir (page 30)

⅛ to ¼ teaspoon spirulina powder

Place the kefir and spirulina into a glass jar, leaving 1 inch (2.5 cm) of space at the top, and put the lid on.

Keep the jar at room temperature and out of direct sunlight for 2 days.

Enjoy right away, or store in an airtight bottle in the refrigerator for up to 1 month.

Yield: 1 cup (235 ml)

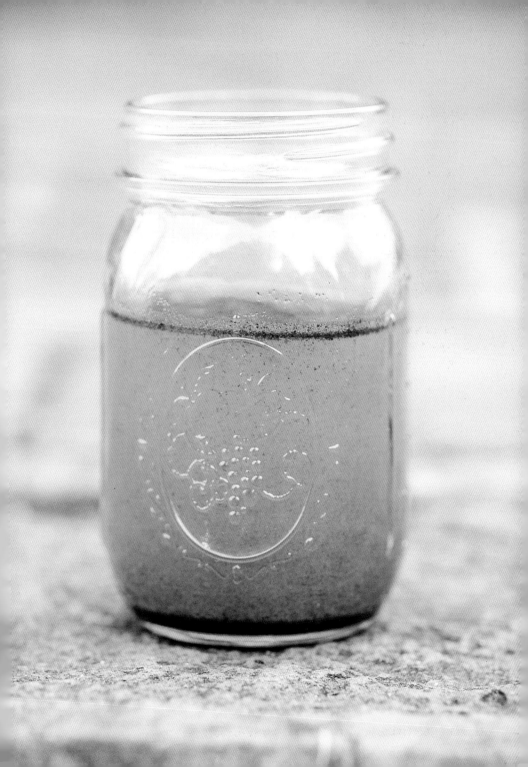

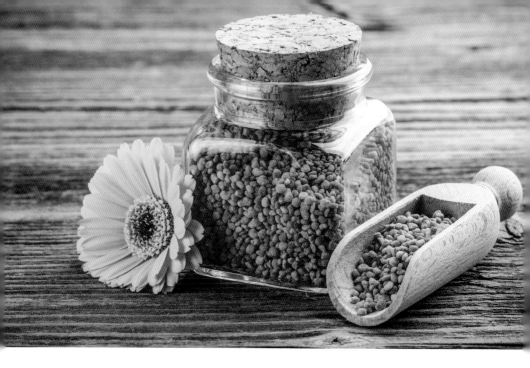

Bee Pollen Kefir

Bee pollen is fabulous! It has a sweet, musky-honey flavor and is loaded with vitamins, minerals, and enzymes. Plus, it has an excellent protein profile. I would love someone to test fermented bee pollen to see whether and how the process enriches its talents even further! Due to the delicate nature of bee pollen and the acidity of fermented kefir, you may find your bee pollen just dissolves into the liquid after a little time. This is completely fine.

1 cup (235 ml) Basic Water Kefir (page 26)

1 teaspoon bee pollen

Place the kefir and bee pollen into a glass jar, leaving 1 inch (2.5 cm) of space at the top, and put the lid on.

Keep the jar at room temperature and out of direct sunlight for 2 days.

Enjoy right away, or store in an airtight bottle in the refrigerator for up to 1 month.

Yield: 1 cup (235 ml)

Antibiotic Repair Kit Smoothie

Honestly, drinking kefir is the best thing that you can do food-wise after a course of antibiotics. And as mentioned earlier in the chapter, it can be beneficial to drink during your course of antibiotics to reduce any symptoms. I have added some extra prebiotics to this smoothie, to assist with the recolonization of the gut.

1 cup (235 ml) Basic Milk Kefir (page 24)

1 banana

2 tablespoons (10 g) rolled oats

1 teaspoon slippery elm powder (optional)

Add all of the ingredients to a blender and blend on high speed until smooth. Enjoy right away.

Yield: 1½ cups (355 ml)

Immunity Kombucha

Jam-packed with immune-boosting vitamin C, this beverage will set you back on the path to wellness.

1 cup (235 ml) Basic Kombucha (page 32)

¼ cup (60 ml) carrot juice

1 tablespoon (15 ml) freshly squeezed lemon juice

Zest of ½ orange (preferably organic)

2 slices fresh ginger (do not peel)

Place the kombucha into a clean glass jar, leaving at least 1 inch (2.5 cm) of space at the top. Add the carrot juice, lemon juice, orange zest, and ginger, and put the lid on.

Keep at room temperature and out of direct sunlight for 1 to 2 days. This will depend on the temperature of your home.

Once this second fermentation is complete, strain out the ginger and zest and transfer your kombucha to an airtight bottle. Store in the refrigerator for up to 1 month.

Yield: 1¼ cups (285 ml)

Carrot Cake Kefir

This is a creamy drink that almost feels a little too naughty to be good for you! There's plenty of protein, good fat, and nutrients in this one, along with some warming spices. If I don't drink it as is, I like to eat it as a dip with slices of apple—yum!

1½ cups (355 ml) Basic Milk Kefir (page 24) or Basic Coconut Milk Kefir (page 28)

¼ cup (60 ml) almond, hemp, or oat milk, or milk of your choice

1 small frozen banana

½ avocado, pitted and peeled

½ cup (55 g) grated carrot

1½ teaspoons tahini

1 teaspoon pure maple syrup

½ teaspoon ground cinnamon

½ teaspoon ground turmeric

½ teaspoon ground ginger

Add all of the ingredients to a blender and blend on high speed until smooth. Enjoy right away.

Yield: 2½ cups (590 ml)

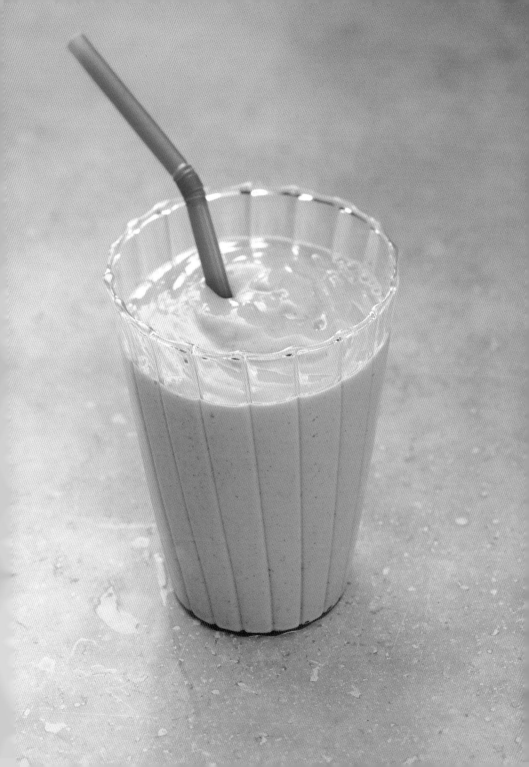

Immunity Supercharger

Make sure you don't need to take that next course of antibiotics by making one of these a regular part of your week. There are huge amounts of vitamin C in this one, which helps prevent and also reduce the length and severity of a cold.

1 cup (235 ml) Basic Water Kefir (page 26)

1 tablespoon (12 g) pomegranate arils

2 slices fresh ginger (do not peel)

Zest of ¼ lemon (preferably organic)

¼ teaspoon ground turmeric or ½ teaspoon sliced fresh turmeric

½ teaspoon herbal hibiscus tea

Place all of the ingredients into a glass jar, leaving 1 inch (2.5 cm) of space at the top, and put the lid on.

Keep the jar at room temperature and out of direct sunlight for 1 to 2 days.

Enjoy right away, or store in an airtight bottle in the refrigerator for up to 1 month.

Yield: 1½ cups (355 ml)

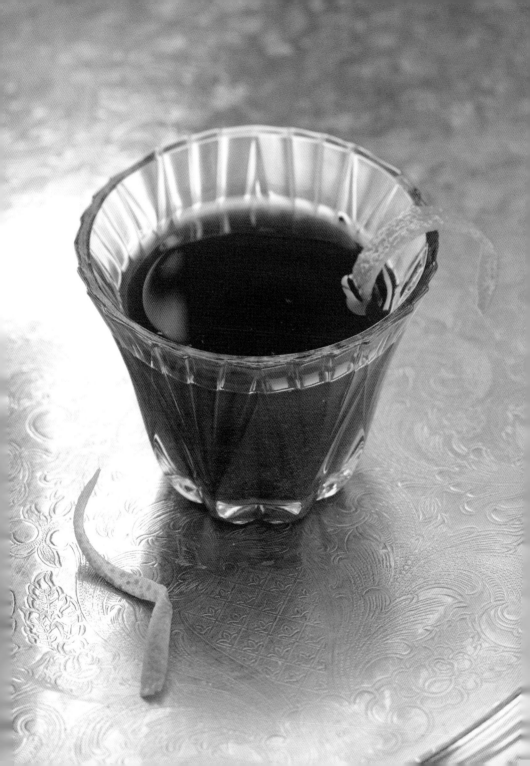

Kiwi Soda

Kiwi is absolutely loaded with vitamin C and is delicious in this lovely, light green soda.

½ cup (120 ml) water, plus more to fill up the bottles

¼ to ¾ cup (50 to 150 g) organic white sugar, to your taste

1 pound (455 g) kiwi, peeled

¼ cup (60 ml) ginger bug or turmeric syrup (page 119)

2 tablespoons (30 ml) freshly squeezed lemon juice

Place a large saucepan on the stove and bring the ½ cup (120 ml) water to a boil. Add the sugar, stirring until dissolved. Stir in the kiwi, then take the mixture off the heat and allow to cool completely.

Transfer the mixture to a blender and blend until smooth.

Push the mixture through a fine-mesh strainer or a nut milk bag to drain out as much of the syrupy juice as you can into a bowl.

Pop the juice into a 1-liter bottle and add water to fill the bottle about two-thirds full. Add the ginger bug starter and the lemon juice, making sure there is still about 1 inch (2.5 cm) of space left at the top.

Allow to sit at room temperature, covered with a piece of cheesecloth to keep the bugs out.

Once your mixture begins to bubble vigorously (this may take a day or a few days depending on the temperature), it is time to cap it and let it sit in a dark place for at least another 2 days to carbonate. Keep checking on your soda, because if you let the carbonation build up too much, your bottle will explode. "Burp" your bottle frequently by loosening the lid and allowing the air to escape, and then replacing the lid.

Once you have reached the carbonation level that you are happy with, drink it, or transfer to the refrigerator to slow down the fermenting process.

Yield: 4¼ cups (1 liter)

Beet Kvass

Kvass is a Russian fermented beverage, traditionally made with rye bread. It is lightly fermented not only to increase the longevity of the drink, but also to provide the usual gamut of benefits such as beneficial microbes, digestive assistance, and bioavailability of nutrients. This beet version sneaks in blood- and liver-cleansing nutrients to boot. And the great thing about this recipe is that you can also use it in place of vinegar in salad dressings or add it to soups. Also, I love to add 1 to 2 ounces (28 to 60 ml) of beet kvass to freshly squeezed vegetable juice such as carrot or beet, and add slices of ginger for an extra kick.

2 large or 3 medium beets (preferably organic)

2¼ teaspoons (15 g) sea salt

Water as needed

Wash the beets to remove any dirt, and slice off any dodgy-looking bits, but do not peel them. Coarsely chop the beets and add to a 2-quart (2-liter) jar. Add the salt and enough water to almost fill the jar. Leave a couple of inches at the top, as the fermenting process will produce carbon dioxide, and you need to give the gorgeous bubbles room.

Allow to ferment at room temperature for 1 to 2 weeks.

Keep in the refrigerator once it has reached a sourness level you are happy with. This drink is supposed to taste quite salty.

Yield: 2 quarts (2 liters)

CHAPTER 3

Cultured Cleansing: Fermented Beverages for Detoxification and Liver Health

Detoxification is a normal and healthy body function—in fact, our body detoxes itself every minute of every day! It is the body's way of creating balance and preventing disease. Sweat, tears, mucus, earwax, fevers, skin breakouts, even sneezing are all channels of elimination for our body to release impurities and maintain healthy function. If a particular organ of the body becomes overburdened, toxins and waste begin to accumulate in our body's tissues. In an effort to maintain balance, the body cleanses itself via one of the above pathways. Toxins from the air we breathe, the food we eat, and the water we drink are transformed and eliminated by the body. Cultured beverages, along with other dietary and lifestyle choices and strategies, have an influential role to play in this process. The problem arises when our bodies become overwhelmed by the amount of toxins they have to deal with.

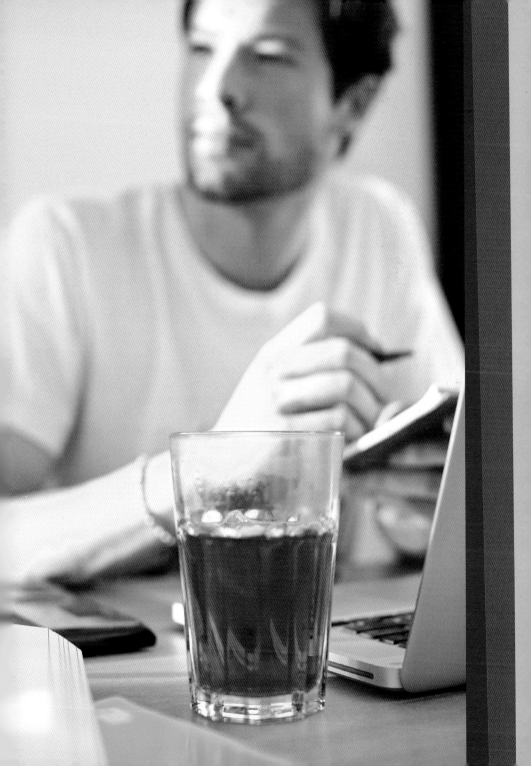

What Are Toxins?

A toxin is a poison of plant or animal origin, especially one produced by or derived from microorganisms and acting as an antigen in the body. Essentially, this means any compound that has a negative effect on cell function. Normally, when we think of toxins, we think of environmental pollution and toxic chemicals. Unfortunately, the list of toxins in our daily life is long and includes many things we probably don't commonly label as toxic, such as alcohol from our nightly glass of wine, caffeine from our daily latte habit, even common prescription and over-the-counter medications. In addition, our air, food, and everyday products such as house cleaners and toiletries are filled with toxins that the body must clear, such as heavy metals, pesticides, herbicides, food additives, and cleaning solvents. By exposing our bodies to these extra toxins, we are creating extra work for our liver and our other organs of elimination.

Toxins are also produced *within* the body from the breakdown of microbial compounds and bacteria and from normal cell functioning. Even the very moment of conception where the egg and sperm meet creates waste by-products that need to be detoxified. Every cell produces normal daily waste, which is then usually picked up by the lymphatic system and processed. The lymphatic system is a collection of vessels that carries fluid (lymph) from our tissues to the blood. An example of this process becoming overwhelmed is when we have a massage. During and after a massage, larger amounts of these waste products are released, and we may experience headaches, fatigue, or general soreness afterward, as the body has to deal with more toxins in circulation than it normally would.

The Liver: Our CEO of Detoxification

The liver is the primary organ responsible for the gigantic task of ridding the body of the toxins that we breathe in, ingest, and put on our skin. What a job! Long hours, cramped work space, constantly picking up the slack from others: Our livers really deserve a holiday.

So how do you know if your liver is overburdened? You may not notice anything to begin with, but after some time the body may send you messages that all is not rosy. Toxins that our body cannot deal with are stored in our tissues, especially our fat cells. It is similar to sweeping the dust under the rug: It's better than being all over the floor, but at some point, we are going to have a problem. The accumulation of toxins in the body can lead to the formation of free radicals, very unstable chemical compounds that can cause damage to our tissues by attacking the DNA and cell membranes. We start to see symptoms such as skin breakouts, headaches, chronic fatigue, nighttime waking, pale stools, nausea, and inflammatory diseases. Fortunately, the liver is amazing, and its function can be improved through diet, lifestyle, and specific nutritional inclusions such as fermented beverages. It can even completely regenerate itself from as little as 25 percent of its tissue!

Other Organs of Detoxification

Thankfully, the liver does have a trusty team of assistants in detoxification. The kidneys are primarily responsible for eliminating metabolic waste, which includes the toxic overload from the breakdown of protein and nucleic acid (for example, DNA) in the body. The bowels are a major route of elimination, and they are also largely involved in the assimilation of nutrients from the food we eat. As food passes along our digestive tract, any usable nutrients are absorbed, and the rest is eliminated via our stools. The lungs and the function of breathing remove carbon dioxide from our body, assisting in maintaining a healthy acid-alkaline balance in our blood. And finally our skin, our largest organ, excretes toxins through sweat.

A Cleansing Lifestyle

We live in quite a toxic world, and given that we can't live in a bubble, it is important to incorporate measures to counteract the effect that exposure to excess toxins has on our bodies. General naturopathic recommendations include eating a plant-based, whole foods diet comprised of organic produce to minimize exposure to pesticides, exercising regularly to aid the body's natural detoxification processes of breathing and perspiring, consuming plenty of fiber and water to speed waste through the kidneys and colon, reducing alcohol and caffeine where possible, and perhaps undertaking regular more structured cleanses, preferably under the supervision of a health care practitioner.

Cultured beverages are an important part of this program, playing a protective and supportive role to the liver and its processes.

How Does Detoxification Work?

There are three primary steps to detoxification performed by the liver. It filters the blood of toxins—up to 99 percent of them when it's functioning at peak performance. It produces bile, which then binds with toxins and carries them out of the body. Finally, the liver converts and excretes toxins via phase I and phase II liver detoxification. During phase I, toxic compounds are put through several processes that improve their water solubility. During phase II, the metabolites are combined with other molecules to render them less active, thus making them easier to transport out of the body. The basic idea is to take the toxin, often a fat-soluble substance, and convert it into a more water-soluble product, so that it can be more easily excreted out of the body instead of stored in our fat cells.

This is why it's important to have all our channels of elimination and detoxification working optimally when we lose weight. When we lose fat, the toxins that have been stored in it are released into the body and can wreak havoc if they are not cleaned up.

Glutathione: The Super Antioxidant

This cleaning process is dependent upon having enough glutathione (GSH). Glutathione is a major antioxidant produced in the body and is available from some foods. GSH helps immune function, reduces inflammation, and protects cells and cell membranes. When we are exposed to toxins, we use up GSH faster than we can produce it and therefore put our bodies in danger of having unbound toxins, known as free radicals, on the loose. These damaging molecules are unstable, as they are missing one electron. They are constantly searching the body for an extra electron so that they can become stable. When they bond with another molecule, they steal one of their electrons and therefore make that previously healthy tissue into another free radical. The process begins again with this molecule having to look for another electron to steal to become stable again. Antioxidants such as GSH help stop this process. Cigarette smoking is a good example of an increased need for GSH. First, the influx of nicotine brings a huge amount of toxic material into the body that needs to be detoxified by GSH and other processes. Second, extra free radicals from the toxins in the smoke need to be stabilized and therefore require more GSH and other antioxidants to get the job done.

Other Important Acids That Aid Detoxification

Certain acids formed during the fermentation of kombucha, such as D-saccharic acid 1,4-lactone (DSL), have amazing antioxidant ability. Research in the *Journal of Chromatography* in 2010 displays the fantastic work of this acid and the way that it inhibits other destructive enzymes whose raison d'etre is to break up beautifully formed bonds of acids and toxins. By breaking up these bonds, the toxins are released back into the blood instead of being safely transported to the liver for proper detoxification and then out of the body.

Kombucha also possesses gluconic acid, which plays two roles in detoxification. First, it binds with heavy metals, assisting to escort them out of the body. Second, gluconic acid supports the work of glucuronic acid, which is a potent natural detoxifier and involved in phase II liver detox.

There are mixed opinions on whether or not kombucha actually contains glucuronic acid, but regardless, it improves the function of glucuronic acid, and liver function in general.

We also require certain nutrients for this whole process to run smoothly, in particular B vitamins and vitamin C, which assist the body to make GSH and complete detoxification pathways. Kombucha not only contains vitamin C and B vitamins, but also the fermenting process makes the vitamins more bioavailable, meaning it is easier for the body to absorb them.

Although we have spoken about kombucha in relation to its benefits for detoxification, a glass of kombucha is much more than a collection of acids, bacteria, and nutrients. It is a complete health tonic, with benefits crossing all spectrums of health, as shown in other chapters of this book. Consuming cultured beverages and foods, in conjunction with a whole foods diet, will bring us great benefits, along with a side of well-being!

Kombucha and Glutathione

GSH is extremely important to the body, and fermented beverages, kombucha in particular, have been shown to protect the body's GSH stores due to their antioxidant status. A study in the *Journal of Biomedical Environmental Science* in 2001 shows kombucha to prevent a drop in GSH levels under conditions of exposure to cold and stress.

In addition to helping out with GSH, kombucha has been found to protect liver cell damage from drugs and other chemicals, including paracetamol (acetaminophen). A 2011 study cited in *Pathophysiology Journal*, and another study in *Comparative Clinical Pathology* in 2012, hypothesized that this is possibly due to the antioxidant activity of kombucha.

Kefir and Detoxification

But it's not just kombucha that is in the spotlight for detoxification. Kefir and its army of good bacteria can also protect the detoxification function of the liver and kidneys. In addition to the benefits we learned about in chapter 1, kefir can help break down and eliminate pesticides. It also appears that kombucha and kefir work better when they are combined. A study in 2010 from the *Journal of Applied Biochemistry and Biotechnology* showed that there was a symbiosis between the microorganisms in kombucha and kefir. This mutually beneficial interaction enhanced the function of kombucha—another win for holistic treatment! This goes back to the idea that it is not one particular strain of bacteria or one component of fermentation that is responsible, but rather a combination of factors working together.

The Benefits of Beets and Beet Kvass

A study in March 2013 in the journal *Phytotherapy Research* showed beetroot to be protective against liver damage, and showed that it improved phase II liver detox and glutathione levels. Another study from 2012 in the journal *Food and Chemical Toxicology* demonstrated beetroot's protective effect on the liver due to the particular antioxidants found within, called betalains. In addition to this wonderful antioxidant profile, beets have traditionally been used to treat liver stagnancy, to purify the blood, and for liver problems in general. This makes beetroot a perfect-combination with any fermented beverage.

Putting It into Practice

- The liver is the primary organ of detoxification, assisted by the kidneys, bowels, lungs, and skin.

- Glutathione is a major antioxidant involved in detoxification. It is necessary to deal with toxins that we are exposed to, and also helps strengthen immune function, reduce inflammation, and protect cells and cell membranes.

- Kombucha assists in detoxification in a number of ways. First, it protects the body's glutathione stores. Second, it protects against liver cell damage and produces antioxidant by-products. Finally, kombucha contains gluconic acid, which binds to heavy metals and carries them out of the body, and also supports the role of glucuronic acid, a potent detoxifier involved in phase II liver detoxification.

Cultured and Fermented Beverage Recipes for Detoxification

Ginger and Turmeric Cleansing Tea

Turmeric is one of my favorite spices. Bright as sunshine, this herb is anti-inflammatory, antioxidant, antimicrobial, and anticarcinogenic. It also stimulates phase II detoxification in the liver. Add relaxing the gut and supporting liver function and you have a very impressive résumé.

2 cups (475 ml) Basic Kombucha (page 32)

2 slices lemon (preferably organic)

1 teaspoon grated fresh ginger (do not peel)

½ teaspoon ground turmeric

Pour the kombucha into a glass jar and add the lemon, ginger, and turmeric. Allow to ferment for 2 to 4 days. Enjoy!

If you don't want to wait, this one works beautifully straight up—combine your kombucha with the rest of the ingredients and drink right away.

Yield: 2 cups (475 ml)

Herbal Detox Tea

Supercharge the already beneficial detoxification effects of kombucha with some detox-specific herbs! Designed to encourage lymphatic clearance and support the kidneys and liver, this combination is particularly useful during a cleanse. It's also great for clearing up the skin.

¾ cup (175 ml) water

½ teaspoon dried calendula

½ teaspoon dried nettle

½ teaspoon dried dandelion leaf

½ teaspoon dried peppermint

¼ cup (60 ml) Basic Kombucha (page 32)

Bring the water to a boil. Combine the herbs in a bowl and pour the boiling water over them. Leave to infuse for 5 to 10 minutes, then strain out the herbs. When cooled to room temperature, add the kombucha and sip slowly.

Yield: 1 cup (235 ml)

The Morning After Smoothie

You are unlikely to make this one in advance, and you would most likely be in need of this in a hurry, without too much thinking involved. What you need on the morning after is alkalinity and some liver assistance, so I have aimed to pack in as much of this as possible! Cucumber is one of the most alkaline vegetables, and it's paired here with the avocado and spirulina for more alkalinity plus B vitamins, good fats, and protein, and apple for added glutathione—this should set you back on the straight and narrow.

⅔ cup (160 ml) water

⅓ cup (80 ml) Basic Kombucha (page 32)

1 (3-inch, or 7.5-cm) piece cucumber

½ green apple (preferably organic)

¼ avocado, pitted and peeled

⅛ to ¼ teaspoon spirulina powder, or as much as you can handle

2 or 3 ice cubes

Place all of the ingredients into a blender, and blend on high speed until smooth. Sip slowly for maximum absorption.

Yield: 1½ cups (335 ml)

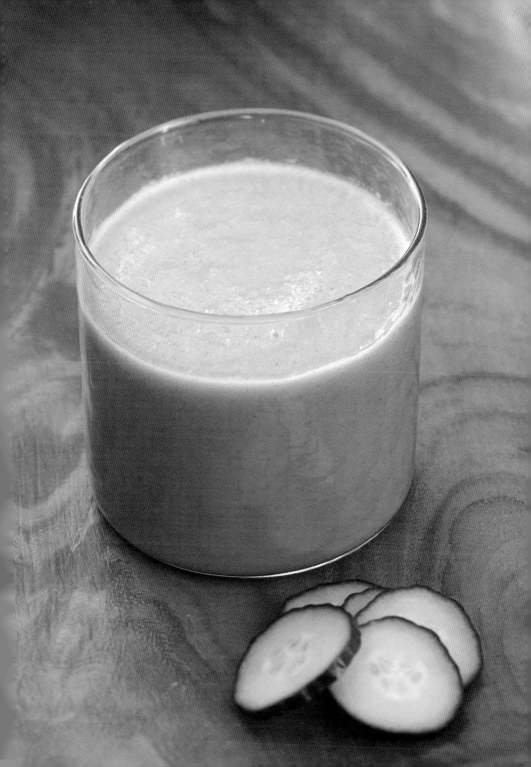

The Overindulger's Tonic

Similar to the Morning After Smoothie on page 82, this tonic is for those who prefer their antidote less viscous. It also has the added electrolyte benefit of coconut water.

⅓ cup (80 ml) Basic Coconut Water Kefir (page 30)

⅓ cup (80 ml) water

1 (3-inch, or 7.5-cm) piece cucumber

¼ green apple (preferably organic)

A good squeeze of lemon or lime juice

4 to 6 fresh mint leaves

¼ to ½ teaspoon peeled and grated fresh ginger

2 or 3 ice cubes

Place all of the ingredients into a blender, and blend on high speed until smooth. Enjoy!

Yield: 1 cup (235 ml)

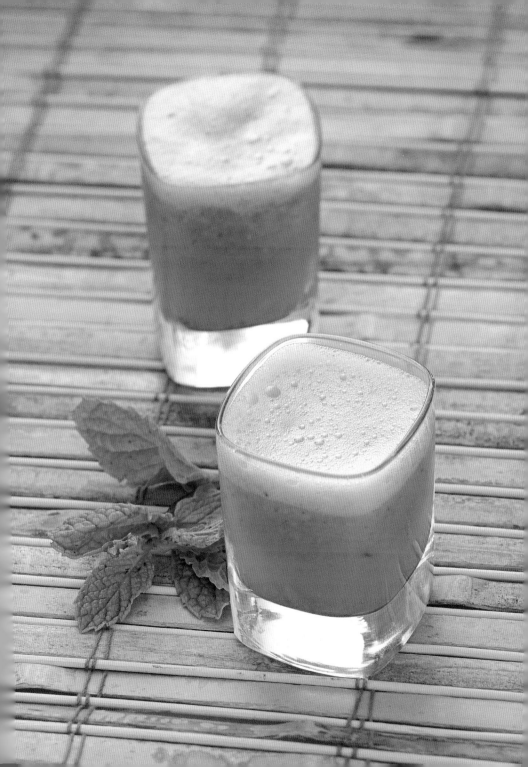

Morning Liver Tonic ▸

Beautifully simple but effective. Lemon gives you the ultimate kick-start to your morning, waking up the digestive system and preparing you for the day ahead.

½ cup (120 ml) Basic Kombucha (page 32)

½ to 1 teaspoon freshly squeezed lemon juice

Pour the kombucha into a teacup. Add the lemon juice to the kombucha, starting with ½ teaspoon and adding a little more if desired. Sip upon waking, before breakfast.

Yield: ½ cup (120 ml)

Spiced Dandelion Tea

Roasted dandelion root is a great friend to the liver, and to digestion in general. It helps the liver produce and release bile, and it is a mild diuretic, meaning that it increases urinary excretion of waste. Its bitterness helps with the release of digestive enzymes to properly digest our food. What a winner!

1 cup (235 ml) Basic Kombucha (page 32)

1 roasted dandelion root tea bag or 1 teaspoon chopped roasted dandelion root

1 cinnamon stick

Pinch of ground nutmeg

Pinch of ground ginger

Pour the kombucha into a jar and add the dandelion tea bag and cinnamon stick. Allow to ferment with the lid on for 1 day at room temperature. Add the nutmeg and ginger, and enjoy!

Yield: 1 cup (235 ml)

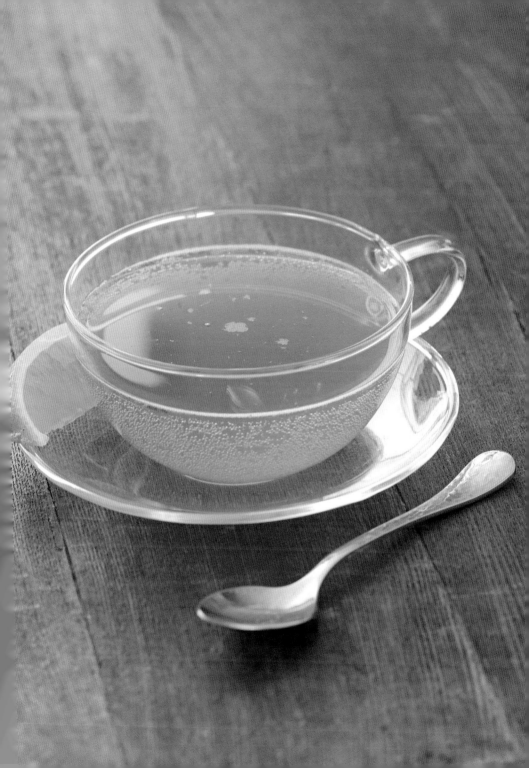

Beet-tastic Kombucha

I adore beets. They are completely underrated, fabulously nutrient rich, and unapologetically messy! There are a number of studies that show beetroot's protective effect on liver cells and also its role in assisting phase II liver detoxification. Beets are fabulous for the liver. They have a wonderful antioxidant profile, and traditionally they have been used to treat liver stagnancy, to purify the blood, and for liver problems in general. Couple that with kombucha, and you have a powerful detoxifying drink that just happens to be refreshing and delicious, too!

1 large beet (preferably organic)

½ cup (120 ml) Basic Kombucha (page 32)

Fresh mint leaves, for serving

Peel the beet and put it through a juicer. You should end up with about ½ cup (120 ml) juice. Combine the beet juice and kombucha in a glass, adorn with some fresh mint leaves, and sit back and enjoy, all aglow in the fact that you have done your good deed for the day—helping out your liver.

Yield: 1 cup (235 ml)

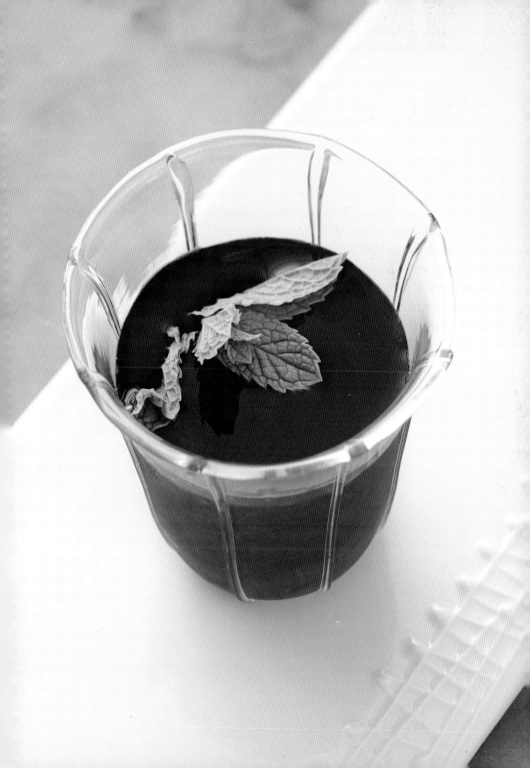

Gingery Beet Kombucha

This little powerhouse is a version of the previous recipe, but with a different brewing process and the addition of ginger. This recipe is fantastic for liver detox and also for when you are feeling a bit under the weather. The ginger will kick-start your circulation, and the nutrient-rich beet will flood your body with antioxidants, iron, potassium, manganese, magnesium, vitamin C, and B vitamins.

½ cup (120 ml) Basic Kombucha (page 32)

¼ cup (56 g) peeled and coarsely chopped beet (preferably organic)

1½ teaspoons finely chopped fresh ginger (do not peel)

Combine all of the ingredients in an airtight jar. Leave at room temperature for 1 to 2 days. Keep checking on your brew, as you will notice bubbles start to form. When it has reached a sourness level that you are happy with, it's ready. Once ready, strain into a clean jar and either enjoy right away or store in the refrigerator for up to 1 month.

Yield: ½ cup (120 ml)

Ginger Beet Kvass

A similar version to the Beet Kvass on page 71, this one includes ginger to offset the salty nature of the drink. It's best sipped in small amounts as a tonic in the morning.

2 large or 3 medium beets (preferably organic)

1 (2-inch, or 5-cm) piece organic fresh ginger, sliced (do not peel)

2¼ teaspoons (15 g) sea salt

Water as needed

Wash the beets to remove any dirt, and slice off any dodgy-looking bits, but do not peel. Coarsely chop the beets and add to a 2-quart (2-liter) jar. Add the ginger and the salt and enough water to almost fill the jar. Leave a couple of inches of space at the top, as the fermenting process will produce carbon dioxide.

Allow to ferment at room temperature for 1 to 2 weeks, until it has reached a sourness level you are happy with. Strain into a clean jar and either enjoy right away or store in the refrigerator for up to 1 month.

Yield: 2 quarts (2 liters)

CHAPTER 4

Culturing a Fertile Body, Healthy Children, and a Healthy Gut from Birth

As babies, we inherit a number of qualities from our parents. Our beautiful blue eyes, our gorgeous freckles—and our gut flora. Yes, among the first gifts passed down from our mothers are the seedlings for a lifetime of bacteria. On our journey through the birth canal into the world, we ingest a good dose of our mother's bacteria, setting up the blueprint for our own individual microbial ecosystem. A study in the *Journal of Pediatric Gastroenterology and Nutrition* in 2004 showed that if mothers were given a probiotic containing *L. rhamnosus* GG during late pregnancy, the infant showed a temporary colonization of the gut with *L. rhamnosus* GG for up to six months. These infants also showed higher levels of *B. breve* at five days of age compared with the placebo group, meaning they were already showing a better-established gut flora colony.

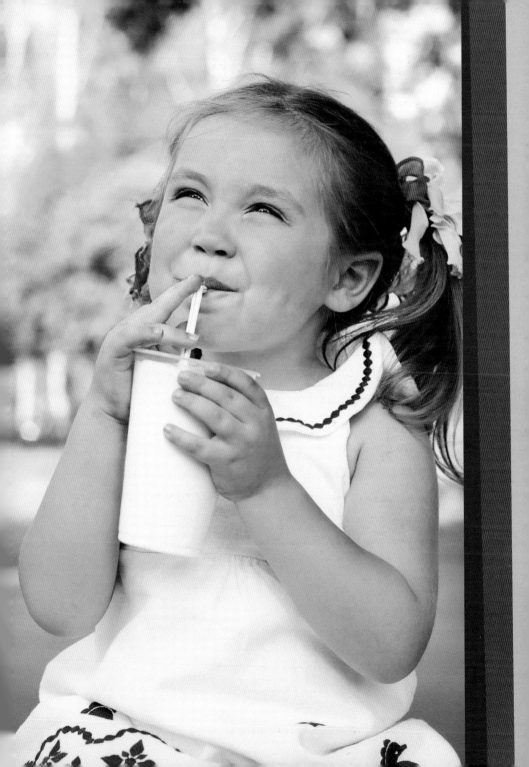

This contact with the mother's bacteria is the first step in creating healthy digestion and immunity for life. It is the quality of this first birthday present that is questionable.

It was originally thought that in the womb, the baby's digestive system was sterile and void of any bacteria. There have recently been some fabulous studies looking at this idea, and finding that the colonization of the digestive tract may begin during our time inside the womb, within the amniotic fluid. An article from the Public Library of Science in 2008 says that the amniotic fluid contains a greater diversity of microbes than previously thought.

This is one important reason to make sure that a mother's gut flora is in prime condition during and preferably before pregnancy. Take your folate, and take your probiotics, whether they be in the form of a powder or fermented drink or food. Sounds easy enough. As we learn more about gut bacteria, it is becoming clearer that the state of the mother's gut potentially influences children's immune system development, the way that they will digest food and absorb nutrients, and their behavior. Given this information, if there are any major issues with gut health, it is important to resolve these prior to pregnancy. The introduction of cultured beverages *before* conception is a fabulous way to address this.

Could Bacteria Influence Time of Birth?

Given that it is normal for babies to swallow 400 to 500 milliliters of amniotic fluid each day, the makeup of this fluid is certainly worth investigating. Initial research seems to be linking preterm labor (delivery before 37 weeks gestation) and the microbial balance in the amniotic fluid. Further research needs to be done, but initial results seem to be indicating a relationship among the type of bacteria, any potential infection within the fluid, and preterm labor. The current thinking, as reported in the *Journal of Clinical Neonatology* in 2011, is that microbes swallowed by the infant in the amniotic fluid where an infection is present may stimulate an inflammatory response, setting off a cascade of events leading to early delivery.

Mother's Gut Flora

During pregnancy, women go through a dramatic hormonal shift. With this influx of extra hormones comes any or all of the following: luscious hair, glowing skin, stronger and faster-growing nails, nausea, constipation, insomnia, and heartburn—ah, the highs and lows of pregnancy. But holding your Hollywood hair out of the way of your morning sickness is not the only new challenge during pregnancy. These hormonal changes have follow-up effects for digestion. Progesterone is one of the main hormones needed to maintain a pregnancy. Levels of progesterone begin to rise from ovulation, reaching a peak toward the end of the cycle. In the case of conception, progesterone levels will remain high, instead of dropping as they do in a normal menstrual cycle. The flip side to this is that progesterone may also create an environment in the body where unhealthy bacteria and yeasts can flourish. The high level of sugars needed for the baby's developing brain creates an acidic environment where certain unruly types of bacteria like to grow. If there is an imbalance of gut flora prior to pregnancy, there is a likelihood that this will be exacerbated during pregnancy.

Why Is It Important to Have Healthy Gut Bacteria in Pregnancy?

Overall intestinal microbiota during pregnancy is associated with cholesterol levels, folic acid, and body weight. A study in the *British Journal of Nutrition* in 2010 showed that in an analysis of stool samples, an increased healthy bacteria level in the guts of pregnant women was related to increased folic acid levels, higher levels of HDL (good) cholesterol, and healthy weight. Given the importance of folic acid levels in particular during pregnancy in the prevention of birth defects, this is fantastic research that should be shouted from the rooftops! A healthy gut equals better levels of folic acid.

Fermented milk containing *Lactobacillus casei DN11401* taken by the mother in the six weeks before delivery and the six weeks after birth increased the mother's immune cells and decreased inflammatory markers in her breast milk, according to a 2008 study in the *British Journal of Nutrition*. The study also showed the children to have fewer gastrointestinal symptoms such as reflux, diarrhea, colic, constipation, and oral thrush compared with the control group.

Another study from the *British Journal of Nutrition* in 2009 analyzed the effect of giving pregnant women two strains of bacteria (*Lactobacillus rhamnosus GG* and *Bifidobacterium lactis Bb12*) along with dietary counseling. The results showed that the women who took the bacteria had a better glucose metabolism, a reduced risk of elevated glucose concentration, and a higher insulin sensitivity in the last trimester of pregnancy compared with the group that received dietary counseling only. This is important, as balanced blood glucose ensures optimal fetal growth and positive health implications for both the mother and the child.

What Can We Do to Optimize Gut Health in Pregnancy?

Fermented beverages are a fabulous addition to any prenatal regime. They will not only work to create the healthy foundation of a balanced gut but can also provide greater access to nutrients via the increased levels of vitamins, in particular B vitamins, that accumulate during the process of fermentation. Minerals also become more bioavailable, and certain compounds are broken down and become easier to digest. For example, the lactose in milk is broken down by lactic acid bacteria into lactic acid, a less reactive and more easily digested compound.

Introduction of fermented beverages *during* pregnancy if you are not already a regular user comes with its cautions. Although there is not a great deal of research on the topic, it is generally recommended that if you don't already consume fermented beverages regularly, pregnancy may not be the ideal time to start. There are a couple of reasons for this.

The detoxification quality of fermented beverages makes them likely to increase the release of toxins into the blood of the mother, to which the baby is then exposed. Detoxification is not recommended during pregnancy, as you are increasing the toxicity of the body for a given time, which the baby then has to handle.

Dr Miin Chan, from the company Doctor Chan's Feeling Good Ferments, explains that women who choose to consume fermented beverages during pregnancy or breast-feeding must be diligent about keeping their hydration levels up to assist with this process.

She also suggests that caution must be exercised with home brewing during pregnancy and breast-feeding, as the complex combination of bacteria and yeasts may potentially pose a risk. There is a very small chance that something may go awry in the fermentation process. Generally in this case, the batch would be discarded and you would begin again. You would not give it to a pregnant woman. If a woman is concerned but still wants to consume home-brewed fermented beverages, Dr. Chan recommends testing your brew with pH strips, which are readily available at pharmacies, to be safe.

Another caveat is that mothers with immune disorders or gestational diabetes should consult their health care practitioner before consuming fermented beverages.

And Dr. Chan suggests that the small amount of alcohol in home-brewed ferments is unlikely to cause a problem, but it is ultimately the mother's choice, in consultation with her physician. She also makes a useful suggestion for breast-feeding mothers to separate their kombucha intake from their breast-feeding session by at least an hour, thus giving any alcohol time to be processed by the liver.

Having said all this, there are some wonderful benefits that fermented beverages can impart during pregnancy. These drinks are consumed in many cultures around the world, and in pregnancy can provide benefits by way of increased energy, better microbial balance, reduction in heartburn, relief from constipation, and increased absorption of vitamins and minerals, says Dr. Chan. Ultimately, it is every woman's own decision, in consultation with her doctor, whether to consume fermented beverages during pregnancy.

Natural versus Caesarean Birth

The business of birth has become quite political of late, and this is not a conversation about that as such. There is no doubt that under normal circumstances, a natural birth is the best way to go for both mother and newborn, given that caesarean birth is related to increased risk for both mother and baby. There is also no doubt that the rate of caesarean births is growing. One study in the journal *Birth* in 2009 reported that in Canada, more than one in four births are performed by caesarean delivery. In the United States, the rate has risen to over 32 percent (National Vital Statistics Report, 2009), in China close to 50 percent (*Lancet*, 2010), and in Brazil 43.9 percent, with this latter percentage reaching 77 percent among those with higher income and who attended a private practice (*Acta Obstetricia et Gynecologica*, 2010).

Aside from an increase in complications for the newborn, caesarean delivery increases the risks of developing asthma, obesity, and type 1 diabetes. One potential explanation for this is gut bacteria. Caesarean-born children are not exposed to the same inoculation of bacteria that is available to newborns as they pass through the birth canal.

An article in *Clinical and Developmental Immunology* in 2013 reports that babies born via caesarean have a delayed development of gut bacteria compared to vaginal-born babies, and they also follow different colonization patterns. First, vaginally born babies have a gut bacteria population after birth that closely resembles their mother's vaginal fluids, while C-section babies have flora that is akin to that of their mother's skin. A study in the *Canadian Medical Association Journal* in 2013 found that compared to vaginally born babies, those born via caesarean had lower numbers of beneficial bacteria, with some (Bifidobacteria) not present at all.

A study in *Applied and Environmental Microbiology* in 2013 explains that Bifidobacteria are a major microbial inhabitant in the infant gut, making up around 60 percent of the total microbial population. This species is thought to assist in the proper development of the baby's immune system, in particular *B. breve*, which assists in the production of serum IgA, the main immunoglobulin involved in protecting the mucosa from pathogens, as described in chapter 2.

The lowest diversity and richness of bacteria was reported from the elective caesarean group, with the highest in the emergency caesarean group. Further research is needed to evaluate whether this is due to partial microbial exposure in the emergency caesarean group.

It is not certain whether diversity and richness of bacteria is the appropriate measure to be using as a marker for good infant gut health, or whether it is more important for infants to have particular strains and combinations present. In fact, we don't really know what the perfectly colonized infant gut should look like. From the research that I have read, it looks like this could be a fluid concept, depending on geographical location and the type of food that the mother consumes prior to birth.

Another exciting area of research is happening in Puerto Rico. According to author and activist Michael Pollan, there is currently a trial assessing the outcome of giving caesarean-born children a nice mouthful of the mother's vaginal fluid manually via a swab directly from the mother's vagina, to kick-start their bacterial microbiome. This is one of the most perfectly simple solutions I have heard, and I sincerely hope it catches on.

How an Infant's Gut Is Colonized

The process of the initial colonization of our digestive system from birth is incredibly complex, and we are still learning about how exactly this occurs. We know that the exposure to the mother's digestive flora in the birth canal lays the foundation for our individual gut microbiome. We also know, as mentioned previously, that there is emerging research suggesting that the developing fetus can be exposed to microorganisms in the amniotic fluid.

Compared with the adult gut, the microbiota that inhabit the infant's intestinal tract is variable and less stable. There are conflicting reports as to the type of bacteria that dominate, with Bifidobacteria being the most represented by several weeks of age, according to the *Journal of Applied and Environmental Microbiology*. The specific composition of the infant's gut is heavily influenced by diet. Whether they are breast-fed or bottle-fed and then what happens when solids are added to the mix months later all have a profound effect on the way that infants' gut bacteria develops and colonizes.

Other factors, such as bacteria from the mother's skin and from the environment, add to the mix, and the potential use of antibiotics by the mother during pregnancy or the infant after birth plays a role.

Infant behavior may also be affected by gut bacteria, in that certain bacteria types present in the gut seem to be connected with colicky behavior. A higher amount of proteobacteria and a lower prevalence of Bifidobacteria and Lactobacilli were significantly related to infants with colic, reports a study published in the *Official Journal of the American Academy of Pediatrics* in 2013. The proteobacteria were found to produce gas and therefore the symptoms and signs of infant colic such as abdominal pain and persistent crying.

Breast Milk: What Is Actually in It?

Traditionally, it was thought that breast milk was sterile of bacteria; however, this is not the case. Recent studies, including one in *Pharmacology Research* in 2013, show that it contains a convenient supply of good bacteria, dominated by lactic acid bacteria and Bifidobacteria and physiological strains of Staphylococci and Streptococci. These bacteria are thought to protect the baby against infection and encourage a healthy development of the immune system. Breast milk is made up of 40 grams per liter of lipids/fat, 8 grams per liter of protein, 70 grams per liter of lactose, and 5 to 15 grams per liter of oligosaccharides/carbohydrates. Early breast milk also contains a large amount of secretory IgA, immune cells, inflammatory mediators, hormones, and growth factors. Add in healthy bacteria to this mix, and you have what is fairly close to liquid gold for babies.

Breast-Feeding Your Baby to Good Gut Health

Bacteria from the mother's gut travels via the enteromammary pathway during late pregnancy and lactation to the mammary glands, and then on to the baby. This is wonderful news for proper inoculation of the infant gut, but on the flip side, it can have negative consequences if the mother's gut health is not in balance. An overgrowth of pathogenic bacteria in the mother's gut can lead to mastitis. This has an effect not only for the infant being exposed to the same pathogenic bacteria, but also for potential problems with breast-feeding, which may then lead to early weaning.

Breast-fed babies seem to have Bifidobacteria as the dominant bacteria in their guts, with a more diverse range of microbes completing the mix with the introduction of solids. Babies who are not breast-fed tend to have an overrepresentation of Peptostreptococcacae and Verrucomicrobiaceae bacteria, the former being the species of *Clostridium difficile*, which is associated with enteric and allergic disease (*Canadian Medical Association Journal*, 2013).

Interestingly, in the first two to three days of life, vaginally born babies will have a population of potentially pathogenic bacteria and a dormant bacteria Ruminococci existing in the gut before the Bifidobacteria and Lactobaccili take over. According to a study in the *American Society for Nutrition* in 2008, the Ruminococci bacteria play a protective role against the growth and spread of pathogenic bacteria, including Clostridium. The particular oligosaccharides in breast milk are perfectly suited to help feed the Ruminococci bacteria, which explains why infants who are not breast-fed often have a much higher count of Clostridium bacteria in their guts. Babies who aren't breast-fed don't fully acquire their colony of Bifidobacteria until six months after birth.

Breast Milk: Not Just for the Baby!

Nutritional science has been searching for an explanation as to why breast milk contains oligosaccharides, a complex carbohydrate that newborns don't have the enzyme to digest. Surely evolution and Mother Nature would not design our first form of nourishment as anything less than perfect? In actual fact, the oligosaccharides are there for the bacteria, not for the baby. As reported in an article in *Clinical and Developmental Immunology* in 2013, they are there to nourish and feed a particular type of Bifidobacteria—*Bifidobacterium infantis*, which assists in the breakdown and digestion of specific oligosaccharides in breast milk and solid food. So this perfect recipe, developed and refined by natural selection, is designed to nourish the child as a probiotic and nourish the microbes as a prebiotic. What a brilliant combination! Recently, companies that make infant formula have begun adding prebiotics and/or probiotics to their products, in light of the mounting evidence of the importance of developing a healthy, properly colonized gut from birth.

What Happens When Breast-Feeding Stops?

When the time comes to introduce solid foods, the microbiota undergo another huge change. According to Ewing and Tucker in their book *The Living Gut*, weaning is another crucial time because the constant benefits of breast milk are removed from the picture, and the numbers of beneficial bacteria decline, along with their positive effects. This leaves an opportunity for pathogenic bacteria to proliferate while the balance of bacteria is established. The introduction of fermented foods can be wonderful soon after this point.

Ferments and Kids

When it comes time to introduce dairy to a child, kefir is a much better first option. A study in *BMC Immunology* in 2008 states that the consumption of fermented milk containing *L. casei* DN-114 001, either by the mother during breast-feeding or by the child after weaning, resulted in an increase in the number of Bifidobacteria in the gut and a decrease in the number of Enterobacteria and Clostridium.

In addition to this, the very nature of kefir is that the lactose has been partially if not completely broken down, making it far more tolerable and easily digested. It also brings with it additional nutrients and immunity-enhancing factors.

Jason Hawrelak, PhD, of Goulds Naturopathica in Hobart, Australia, agrees that kefir is an ideal first dairy food to introduce when the time comes. The only thing to consider is the fact that kefir is a much more tart-tasting beverage than milk. You can sweeten it with a little banana or berries, but the sourness is not necessarily a bad thing. Exposing children to the slightly sour tastes of fermented foods may help them develop a fully rounded palate, rather than one geared completely toward the sweet and the salty.

Water kefir (tibicos) is another fabulous child-friendly option. It is relatively sweet and slightly fizzy, and it can be enhanced with favorite fruits and other flavors.

In terms of kombucha and children, you should consider the fact that kombucha is typically made from black tea, which contains caffeine. Finished kombucha contains very little caffeine; see the FAQs on page 178. You may choose not to give it to your child for this reason, or you may prefer for your child to have a natural product as opposed to soft drinks and other less natural options. It is every parent's individual decision as to which fermented drinks are right for his or her child.

Putting It into Practice

- We inherit our gut bacteria, and the first contact with our mother's microbiota while passing through the birth canal sets up healthy digestion and immunity for life.

- The health of the mother's gut potentially influences the child's immune system development, the way that the child will digest food and absorb nutrients, and even the child's behavior.

- Pregnant women who have increased levels of healthy bacteria are shown to have increased folic acid levels, higher levels of good cholesterol, and healthy weight.

- Women who supplement with probiotics during pregnancy and after birth tend to have children with fewer digestive complaints.

- Whether infants are breast-fed or bottle-fed and then what happens when solids are introduced has a profound effect on the way that their gut bacteria develops and colonizes.

Cultured and Fermented Recipes for Ensuring a Healthy Gut from Birth

Raw Cultured Almond Coconut Milk with Spiced Chocolate

This is probably my favorite recipe in the book—and it is *very* hard to pick favorites. The spiced chocolate mixture that flavors the milk is absolutely *divine* and will flavor any milk drink beautifully. The almond and coconut combination is full of protein and electrolytes to nourish and replenish. This recipe is lovely with dairy milk kefir also, if you would prefer.

1 cup (145 g) raw unsalted almonds

Squeeze of lemon juice

2 cups (475 ml) coconut water

1 tablespoon (15 ml) Basic Water Kefir (page 26) or Basic Coconut Water Kefir (page 30)

2 teaspoons Spiced Chocolate Mix (recipe follows)

Spiced Chocolate Mix

2 tablespoons (10 g) unsweetened coconut flakes

1 tablespoon (8 g) raw cacao nibs

2 teaspoons vanilla powder

½ teaspoon orange zest

¼ teaspoon ground ginger

Grind up all of the ingredients in a mortar and pestle, coffee grinder, or small blender. Store in an airtight jar in the refrigerator.

Makes 2 heaping tablespoons (20 g)

Soak the almonds overnight at room temperature in a bowl with water and a squeeze of lemon juice. Rinse well and drain.

Add the almonds and coconut water to a blender and blend on high speed until smooth. Strain through a nut milk bag, a fine-mesh strainer, or a piece of cheesecloth, squeezing out as much milk as you can. Set aside the pulp and use to add to cookie or other baking recipes in place of almond meal. Transfer the milk to a clean glass jar or a bowl with a 2-cup (475-ml) capacity. Add the kefir.

Place the spiced chocolate mix in a tea ball, or enclose it in a piece of cheesecloth and tie it with a piece of kitchen string. Place into the almond milk mixture and leave at room temperature for 6 to 8 hours, or until soured to your liking.

Drink right away or store in an airtight bottle in the refrigerator for up to 1 week.

Yield: 2 cups (475 ml)

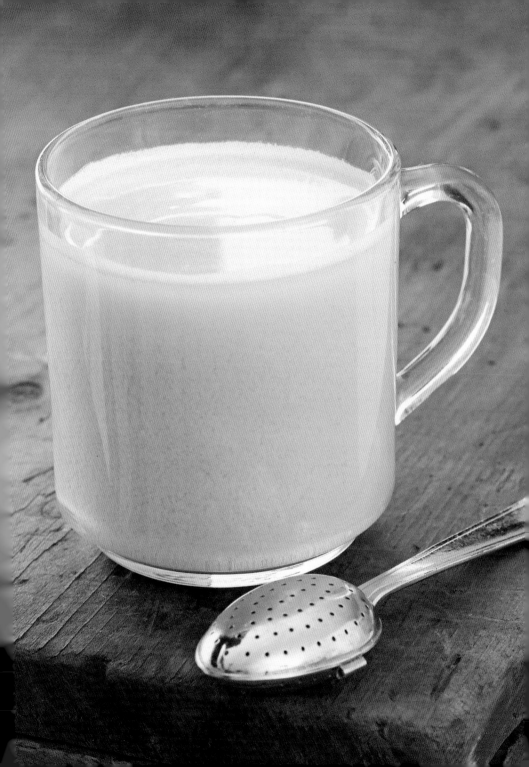

Fermented Strawberry Chia Drink

There are a few chia and kombucha drinks around, so I thought it would be good to have a DIY recipe. You can adjust the amount of chia depending on how thick you like it, and you can use almost any culturing medium. Chia seeds are wonderfully high in protein, minerals, and essential fatty acids. For this recipe, I have kept the chia seeds whole; however, to get the most nutrition out of them, they should be ground. Feel free to grind all or half the seeds in this recipe before soaking, if you like.

¼ cup (50 g) chia seeds

1 cup (235 ml) water

2 cups (475 ml) Basic Kombucha (page 32) or any of the basic kefirs (pages 24 to 30)

½ cup (75 g) fresh or frozen strawberries (preferably organic)

⅓ vanilla bean, split

Soak the chia seeds in the water for 10 minutes, to let the chia absorb the water.

Place the kombucha or kefir into a glass jar and add the soaked chia seeds, strawberries, and vanilla bean. Seal the jar and leave at room temperature for up to 1 day. Strain out the strawberries and vanilla bean and give the mixture a stir. Enjoy as is, or feel free to blend with an immersion blender or in a standing blender if you don't want the chia seeds whole in your drink.

Yield: 2 cups (475 ml)

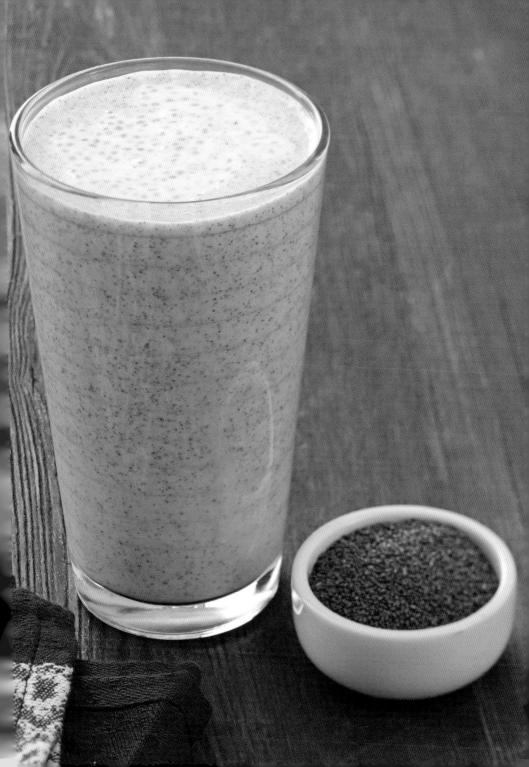

Superfoods Kombucha

This ferment is packed with superfood goodness. Not only does it have the general fabulousness of kombucha, but it also has maca root powder (an energizing superfood powder; see page 160 for more information) for added energy; acai berry powder for an antioxidant boost; and chia for extra protein, fiber, and minerals. It's the perfect pick-me-up!

2 tablespoons (25 g) chia seeds

6 tablespoons (90 ml) water

2 cups (475 ml) Basic Kombucha (page 32)

1 teaspoon maca powder

1 teaspoon acai berry powder

3 or 4 slices lemon (preferably organic)

Soak the chia seeds in the water for 10 minutes, to let the chia seeds absorb the water.

Add all of the ingredients to a glass jar and leave sealed at room temperature for 2 days. Enjoy right away or transfer to an airtight bottle and store in the refrigerator for up to 1 week.

Yield: About 2¼ cups (535 ml)

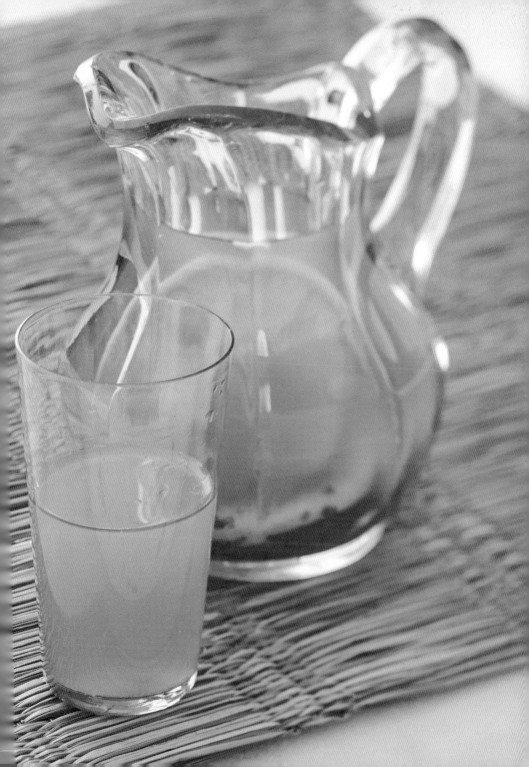

Fertility Smoothie

As discussed, balancing your gut health is vital for ensuring healthy immune and digestive function in your developing baby. This is a preconception smoothie that includes lots of lovely fats, which are necessary to balance hormones and for the development of the child.

1½ cups (355 ml) Basic Coconut Water Kefir (page 30) or Basic Water Kefir (page 26)

¼ to ½ avocado, pitted and peeled

1 frozen banana

½ cup (15 g) spinach leaves

3 tablespoons (38 g) chia seeds

3 tablespoons (45 ml) freshly squeezed lemon or lime juice

6 fresh mint leaves, or more to taste

½ teaspoon spirulina powder (optional)

Place all of the ingredients in a blender and blend on high speed until smooth. Your smoothie will have a thick consistency that you can eat with a spoon! If you would like it thinner, add extra kefir or water to reach the desired consistency. Serve right away.

Yield: 2 cups (475 ml)

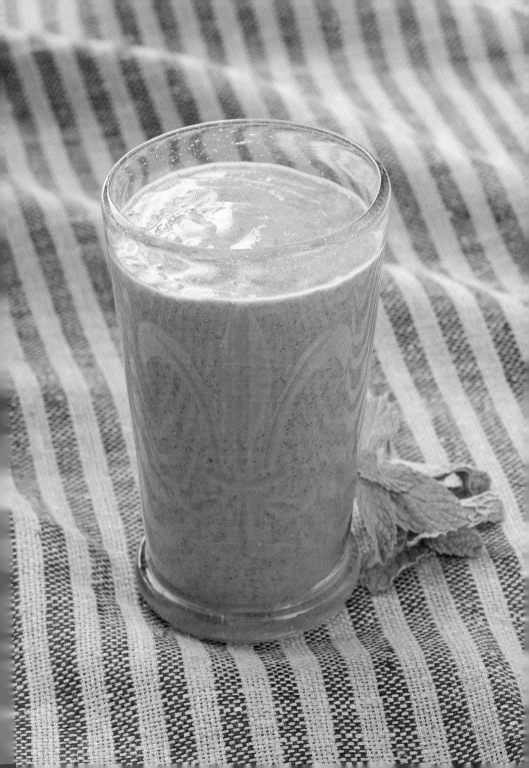

Breast-Feeding Mother's Tonic

This recipe uses quinoa, which is wonderfully high in protein and contains minerals such as magnesium and iron. The coconut water is full of natural electrolytes to replenish the body of nutrients that are lost through the constant burning of calories by breast-feeding. To serve it, add a pinch of cinnamon and a little honey and drink it on its own, or mix it into a smoothie with berries, banana, or coconut milk.

½ cup (86 g) quinoa

Squeeze of lemon juice

1 cup (235 ml) coconut water

1 tablespoon (15 ml) Basic Water Kefir (page 26) or a pinch of kefir starter

Place the quinoa in a bowl and cover with water. Add a squeeze of lemon juice and leave at room temperature overnight covered with a clean kitchen towel.

Drain and rinse the quinoa a couple of times. This rinses off the saponins and prevents it from being too bitter.

Transfer the quinoa to a blender with the coconut water and blend until smooth.

Strain the mixture through a nut milk bag or a piece of fine cheesecloth, squeezing out all the milk that you can.

Pour the milk into a clean jar, and add the finished kefir. Cover with cheesecloth and a rubber band and keep at room temperature for 12 to 24 hours, until it reaches the desired sourness. Just keep tasting it to test. There may be some separation of the milk; this is normal, so if it happens, just give it a good stir.

Yield: 1 cup (235 ml)

Berry Rooibos Kombucha Spider with Kefir Ice Cream

This takes me back to being a kid. My parents would take us out for special occasions and my sister and I would order these crazy iridescent blue ice cream sodas (we call them spiders or floaters in Australia) from a cool inner-city café. I have no idea what was in them . . . well, actually, I do: sugar, and a lot of blue food dye. But we loved them.

So, I have recreated our childhood drink, without the food dye and with minimal sugar but with just as much excitement, if you ask me! The ice cream is a whole food: full-fat, delicious, unapologetic ice cream. It is a treat, and so we shouldn't have to water it down with low-fat versions and fake sugars. Enjoy it in all its glory (in moderation)! I adapted the ice cream recipe from cheeseslave.com. For extra probiotic goodness, you can culture the cream in the same way you make the milk kefir.

½ cup (120 ml) heavy cream

½ cup (120 ml) Basic Milk Kefir (page 24)

½ cup (170 g) honey or pure maple syrup, or more depending on taste

2 egg yolks

½ teaspoon pure vanilla extract or ½ vanilla bean, seeds scraped out

Small pinch of sea salt

2 cups (475 ml) Raspberry Rooibos Kombucha (page 116)

Combine the cream, kefir, maple syrup, egg yolks, vanilla, and salt in a bowl and whisk together. Chill as needed and process in an ice cream maker according to the manufacturer's instructions.

To serve, add 1 cup (235 ml) Raspberry Rooibos Kombucha to 2 tall glasses. Add a scoop of ice cream and serve with a straw and a long spoon!

Yield: Serves 2

Creamy Chocolate Kefir Milk Shake ▸

For those who are not sold on the taste of milk kefir, this is a great way to have it! Great for kids and adults alike, this indulgent-tasting milk shake is full of goodness and contains only three ingredients. It's also sugar-free.

2 cups (475 ml) Basic Milk Kefir (page 24)

2 small frozen bananas

2 tablespoons (12 g) raw cacao powder

Add all of the ingredients to a blender and blend on high speed until smooth.

Enjoy right away, or store in an airtight bottle in the refrigerator for up to 2 days.

Yield: 2½ cups (570 ml)

Kids' Kefir Smoothie

The taste of milk kefir is often quite strong for little ones. You can either brew it for a shorter time to help with the sourness issue, or work it into smoothies like this. I have included lovely fat and protein for their growing bodies. You may substitute sunflower seeds for the almonds in this recipe, if you like.

2 cups (475 ml) Basic Milk Kefir (page 24) or Basic Coconut Milk Kefir (page 28)

1 cup (145 g) berries of your choice (preferably organic)

1 banana

¼ cup (8 g) spinach leaves

¼ cup (35 g) raw unsalted almonds

1 tablespoon (15 ml) pure maple syrup (optional)

Add all of the ingredients to a blender and blend until smooth. Serve right away.

Yield: 3 cups (690 ml)

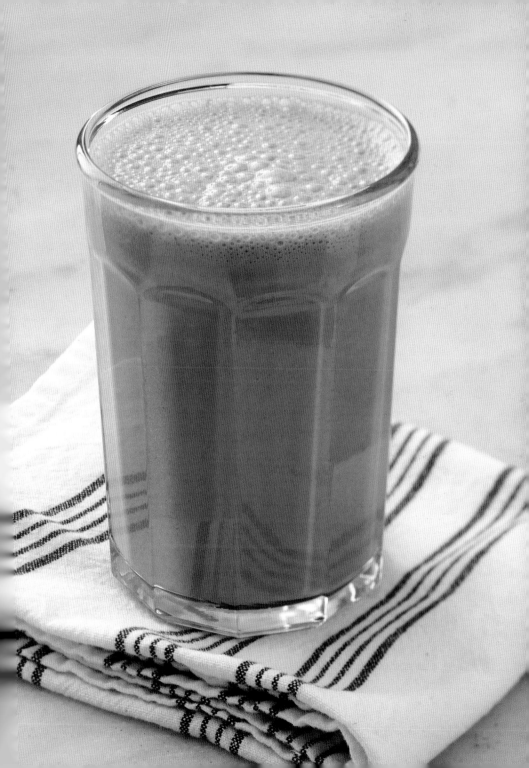

Strawberry and Vanilla White Tea Kombucha

This is a fresh and fruity drink that has a heady note of strawberry along with the delicious muskiness of vanilla. It's perfect for a summer picnic.

2 cups (475 ml) Basic Kombucha (page 32) made with white tea instead of black tea (be sure not to let it go too sour)

½ cup (75 g) strawberries (preferably organic)

½ vanilla bean, split

Fresh mint leaves, for serving

Place all of the ingredients in a glass jar and leave at room temperature for 1 to 2 days.

Strain out the strawberries and vanilla bean and enjoy right away, or store in an airtight bottle in the refrigerator for up to 1 month. Serve over ice with mint. Delicious!

Yield: 2 cups (475 ml)

Raspberry Rooibos Kombucha

Rooibos is a traditional South African herb that has fantastic antioxidant potential—you can read more about it on page 157. It is caffeine-free and adds a lovely mild, smoky-sweet undertone to your kombucha. Mixed with raspberries, this is too delicious!

2 cups (475 ml) Basic Kombucha (page 32) made with rooibos tea instead of black tea

¼ cup (33 g) fresh or frozen raspberries (preferably organic)

Once your rooibos kombucha is brewed to your liking, transfer to an airtight jar and add the raspberries. Leave with the lid on at room temperature for 2 days.

Strain out the raspberries and enjoy right away, or store in an airtight bottle in the refrigerator for up to 1 month.

Yield: 2 cups (475 ml)

Gingerbread Kefir

This is a delicious, festive soda that also has wonderful warming, digestive qualities. Play around with the spice quantities until you reach the perfect mix for your taste preference.

4¼ cups (1 liter) Basic Water Kefir (page 26) or Basic Coconut Water Kefir (page 30)

2 teaspoons Gingerbread Spice (recipe follows)

¾ to 1 teaspoon blackstrap molasses

Add all of the ingredients to a glass jar, leaving 1 inch (2.5 cm) of space at the top. Leave to ferment with the lid on at room temperature for 1 day.

Strain out any larger pieces of spice and enjoy!

Yield: 4¼ cups (1 liter)

Gingerbread Spice

¾ teaspoon ground cinnamon

¾ teaspoon ground ginger

¼ teaspoon ground allspice

¼ teaspoon ground nutmeg

Pinch of ground cloves

Mix all of the ingredients together in a small bowl.

Makes 2 teaspoons

Ginger Beer

To make traditional ginger beer, you first need to make a "ginger bug." This is effectively the starter culture that you will use to culture the drink, as opposed to a SCOBY or kefir grains. The ginger bug can also be used as a starter for other fermented beverages (see pages 70, and 147), or other starters can be used to make the ginger beer, such as water kefir or whey.

4¼ cups (1 liter) water

1 (1-inch, or 2.5-cm) piece fresh ginger (do not peel), thinly sliced, or more to taste

½ cup (100 g) organic white or rapadura (panela) sugar

¼ cup (60 ml) ginger bug (see below)

1 tablespoon (15 ml) freshly squeezed lemon juice

Pour half of the water into a saucepan and add the sliced ginger. Bring to a boil and then simmer for 15 minutes. Take the mixture off the heat, add the sugar, and stir to dissolve. Add the remaining water. Once the mixture has completely cooled, transfer to a wide-mouth jar for fermenting. Pour in the ginger bug, leaving the gingery sediment behind. Add the lemon juice and give the mixture a good stir.

Cover with cheesecloth and a rubber band and leave to ferment at room temperature until the mix becomes bubbly. This may take anywhere from 1 day to several days or longer, depending on the room temperature and the potency of your starter. Once the mix is bubbly, you can bottle it in an airtight 1-liter bottle. The longer you leave it before bottling, the more alcoholic the brew will be. Let the bottle stand at room temperature until carbonated. This usually takes around 14 days, but it may be shorter or longer. Be careful, and check on your bottle frequently, because if you let your bottle over-carbonate, you will have exploding sticky ginger beer all over your laundry

(I speak from experience). Once carbonated, you can refrigerate your ginger beer, which will slow down the carbonation, but it will still continue to pressurize, so continue to check regularly.

How to Make a Ginger Bug

Ginger bugs are one of my favorite things to make. They are so easy and rewarding as you see your little friend bubbling away.

Place ¾ cup (175 ml) water into a small glass jar and add 1 teaspoon organic white or rapadura (panela) sugar and 1 teaspoon grated fresh ginger. Do not peel the ginger, as it is the skin of the ginger that contains all the wonderful yeasts and bacteria that are going to ferment your drink.

Give the mixture a stir, cover with cheesecloth and a rubber band, and leave at room temperature for 1 day.

Add another 1 teaspoon sugar and 1 teaspoon ginger to the mixture and stir well. Keep adding sugar and ginger to the bug each day, stirring frequently, until your mix produces some decent bubbles. If this hasn't happened in 7 days, throw it out and start again. Sandor Katz in his book *The Art of Fermentation* states that a failure to produce bubbles may be due to the fact that the ginger has undergone irradiation, which destroys the bacteria and yeasts. Choose organic ginger for best results.

To make a new ginger bug after use, throw away half of the gingery sediment that is left, add another ¾ cup (175 ml) water, and continue to feed it with 1 teaspoon each of sugar and ginger each day.

How to Make Turmeric Syrup

This variation follows the ginger bug recipe almost exactly. Just use grated fresh turmeric (do not peel) instead of ginger, and follow the same procedure. Once you reach the bottling stage, there is no need to leave the bug to carbonate, as your syrup is ready to use. The resulting fermented syrup can be mixed with fizzy or still mineral water or used in cocktails.

You may, however, leave it to carbonate into a sparkling turmeric beer, using the same procedure outlined in the ginger beer recipe. Delicious!

Yield: 4¼ cups (1 liter)

White Peach and Lavender Soda

This is a lovely summertime soda that is a little bit fancy but not too pretentious. Peaches are so enticing; combine them with a bit of relaxing flower power from the lavender and you have a winning combination. Make sure you use food-grade lavender that has not been sprayed.

½ cup (120 ml) water, plus more to fill up the bottles

¼ to ¾ cup (50 to 150 g) organic white sugar, depending on taste

1 pound (455 g) fresh or frozen peaches, coarsely chopped

¼ cup (60 ml) ginger bug or turmeric syrup (page 119)

3 tablespoons (45 ml) freshly squeezed lemon juice

1 teaspoon fresh unsprayed lavender flowers

Bring the ½ cup (120 ml) water to a boil in a large saucepan. Add the sugar, stirring until dissolved. Stir in the peaches, cook for a few minutes, and then take the mixture off the heat and allow to cool completely.

Place the mixture into a fine-mesh strainer or nut milk bag and apply gentle pressure to drain out as much of the syrupy juice as you can into a small bowl.

Pour the juice into a 1-liter bottle and add water until it reaches 2 to 3 inches (5 to 7.5 cm) from the top. Add the ginger bug, lemon juice, and lavender, making sure there is still about 1 inch (2.5 cm) of space left at the top. Cover and gently shake to distribute the bug, flowers, and juice throughout.

Allow to sit at room temperature covered with a piece of cheesecloth. Once your mixture begins to bubble vigorously (this may take a day or a few days, depending on the room temperature), it is time to cap it and let it sit in a dark place for at least another 2 days to carbonate. Keep checking on your soda, because if you let the carbonation build up too much, your bottle will explode. Burp your bottle frequently by loosening the lid and allowing the air to escape, and then replace the lid.

Once you have reached the carbonation level that you are happy with, drink it, or transfer to the refrigerator to slow down the fermenting process.

Yield: 4¼ cups (1 liter)

Sweet Potato Soda

I first read about a sweet potato drink, traditional to Guyana, in Africa, in *Nourishing Traditions* by Sally Fallon. And it is on that recipe that this one is based. This is a fabulous soda to make for parties or a get-together with friends. It incorporates a sterilized eggshell. This is to provide minerals for the starter and also to neutralize the sourness.

½ large sweet potato

4¼ cups (1 liter) water

½ cup (100 g) organic rapadura (panela) sugar

2 tablespoons (30 ml) Basic Water Kefir (page 26), ginger bug (page 119), or whey (page 173)

Zest and juice of ½ lemon

1 teaspoon ground nutmeg

1 whole clove

Pinch of ground cinnamon

½ eggshell, sterilized (page 27) and crushed

Peel and grate the sweet potato. Place into a colander and rinse under running water until it runs clear to remove the starch. Press out any excess water.

Place the sweet potato, along with all of the other ingredients, into a large bowl and cover with cheesecloth. Leave at room temperature for 2 to 3 days, until the mixture is bubbly.

Pour through a fine-mesh sieve into an airtight bottle and store in the refrigerator.

Yield: 4¼ cups (1 liter)

CHAPTER 5

Culturing for Radiant Skin and a Healthy Mind

Naturopathic philosophy says that the gut is the center of health. It is one of the first things formed as we are developing in the womb and is integral not only to our digestion, but also to our immune system, skin, and brain function. Digestion and immunity we have discussed already, but the gut and its bacteria also have a close relationship with the skin (gut-skin axis) and the brain. For a few years now we have been aware of the link between the brain and the gut (the brain-gut axis); however, new research has highlighted the idea that the connection flows in the opposite direction also, from the gut to the brain. This is a really exciting area of research that is currently being explored, and it illustrates the importance of good gut health and proper balance of microbiota more than ever. First, let's investigate the relationship between the gut and the skin.

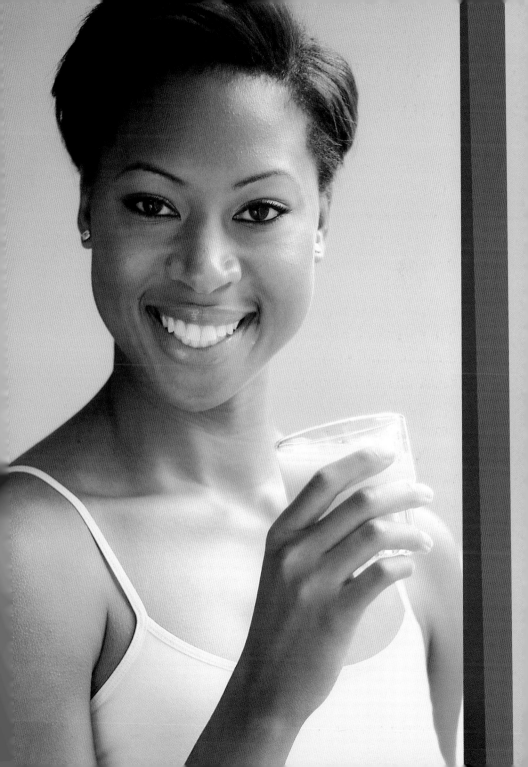

Glowing Skin and Healthy Hair

There is no doubt that we are attracted to glowing skin and shiny, healthy hair. It is a universally recognized sign of good health. Cosmetic and hair product companies have made their living from it. But we are not just attracted to shiny hair and glowing skin because the TV commercial tells us we should be. From an evolutionary standpoint, radiant skin and shiny hair would signal a good choice for reproductive partner, as these qualities are also said to correlate with peak reproductive fitness, which occurs around the age of twenty-five years. It certainly doesn't work that way today, but healthy skin and hair remain a marker for good health. A lot of nutrients and good fats are required to grow healthy skin and hair, so it is a fairly good yardstick to use to judge general health. Also, if we are stressed, tired, or have gone a little crazy on the caffeine and sugary refined foods, our skin can often look dull, dry, irritated, or blemished. The skin is the largest organ in the body, and even though it may appear to be just a fancy covering for our bones, it is a living, breathing, fully functioning organ.

So, we can spend a fortune on skin products and hair treatments, or we can consume probiotics and cultured beverages! Okay, perhaps it is not that simple, but there is some fabulous research emerging about the cosmetic benefits of good gut health.

Probiotics: The New Solution to Dull Skin and Hair Loss?

A study published in the *Public Library of Science* in 2013 tells of their research with probiotic supplementation and the health of skin and hair. Probiotic supplementation with the *L. reuteri* strain, either on its own or in yogurt, showed an increase in hair growth and shine, an increase in skin thickness, and a general "healthful glow." It seems that the probiotic increased the sebocytes, which are the cells that produce sebum, an oily substance that helps prevent skin and hair from drying out. The more sebum that was present, the shinier the hair and more glowing the skin. Also, tissues of those consuming the probiotic supplement were more acidic. Acidic pH is known to alter the hair cuticle and contribute to shiny hair. By improving the bacteria in our gut with fermented beverages, we encourage a more acidic environment, leading to shiny hair and radiant skin. If there were a pharmaceutical drug that could claim to do this, it would be marketed to within an inch of its life. So it is very exciting and encouraging to see this research being done.

Further research in 2011 in the *Proceedings of the National Academy of Sciences* found that an acidic vaginal pH correlated with an abundance of Lactobacillus bacteria and peak fertility in women. Putting these two studies together, we can extrapolate that the probiotic bacteria encourage physiological changes, including a more acidic pH in the body, leading to shiny hair and glowing skin. The fact that this is most likely to occur around the age of twenty-five, peak fertility, is another way Mother Nature has it all organized in a neat little package for us. Given these findings, it would be very interesting to research whether an improvement in gut bacteria could assist fertility in general.

Gut Bacteria Is Sexy!

The other amazing finding from the 2011 *Proceedings of the National Academy of Sciences* study was an increased level of oxytocin released with the intake of probiotics. Oxytocin, produced during kissing and intercourse, is often called the feel-good hormone, as it reduces stress and encourages bonding. This research is in its early days, but it is just fabulous to consider the wide-reaching applications of probiotics, fermented beverages, and good gut health! This, coupled with the glossy hair and radiant skin, is an excellent argument for the sexiness of gut bacteria.

Beautiful Skin with Fermented Beverages

Beneficial effects on the skin using fermented beverages have been noted in several research studies. Certain metabolites of unhealthy gut bacteria called phenols disturb the way that skin cells replicate and divide themselves, and also cause skin dryness. One study in the journal *Beneficial Microbes* in 2013 showed that fermented milk drinks reduced the total phenol levels and prevented skin dryness and disruption of the skin cell replication in adult women.

More exciting still is that a study in 2012 in *Annals of Microbiology* found that two strains of bacteria (*Lactobacillus rhamnosus* FTDC8313 and *Lactobacillus gasseri*

FTDC8131) are capable of producing hyaluronic acid. You have most likely heard about hyaluronic acid in skin care product marketing campaigns, as it is often an ingredient in such products. Itseffects include improved wound healing and tissue repair of the skin, and it plays a role in the maintenance of skin elasticity and correct cell proliferation.

But we aren't yet finished with our fermented beauty school. Fermented beverages also contain lactic acid, which is a natural form of alpha hydroxy acid (AHA), another popular addition to many anti-wrinkle treatments. AHA promotes collagen formation and the production of skin cells and helps reduce the signs of aging. How wonderful that we have access to this via fermented beverages.

The effect that lactic acid has on certain skin conditions is another wonderful side effect of fermented beverage consumption. An article in the *Journal of Dairy Science* in 2006 describes fermented milk's benefits in skin hydration and elasticity, via its ability to increase certain factors in the skin that contribute to skin hydration.

We have already learned about the idea that fermented beverages and probiotics may reduce a child's susceptibility to allergies, but the good news continues in that they can also help reduce the symptoms of atopic dermatitis and eczema in people of all ages. A study in the journal *Gastroenterology in North America* in 2012 found that good gut bacteria and the use of probiotics can alleviate systemic and local allergic inflammation. Healthy gut microbiota teach the immune system to differentiate between pathogenic bacteria and harmless antigens and how to respond appropriately.

Fermented beverages have a role to play here in providing and encouraging the growth of good bacteria, as well as nourishing and assisting with healing of the gut wall. We cannot claim that drinking fermented drinks will *cure* allergies, eczema, and dermatitis. What we can extrapolate, though, is that fermented beverages provide healthy bacteria and further beneficial effects that assist in the healing and nourishing of the digestive system. In this way, not only do they aid in moderating the allergic response, but they also work to heal the gut, which in the long term is the best approach for alleviating symptoms and reducing the expression of the allergic reaction or skin condition.

A Healthy Gut Is a Healthy Mind

It seems that there may be somewhat of a global epidemic emerging in relation to mental heath and depression. Research published in *Health Affairs* in 2003, taking into account data from the United States, Canada, Netherlands, Chile, and Germany, found that up to one-third of all visits to primary care physicians involve emotional disorders such as depression and anxiety. Can we just blame our modern, stress-fueled lifestyles? The cause runs much deeper and is more complex than that. Certainly the urbanization of our lives is a major factor—socioeconomic issues, an increase in sedentary behavior, lack of daily sunlight, lack of face-to-face social connection and support, changes in our diet toward more processed food, and a move away from being connected with the land and with nature. These all play interweaving roles.

An exciting and rapidly growing area of research is the connection between our gut microbiota and our mind. This comes from an understanding that the body functions not as a collection of separate organs, but rather as a whole being whose parts are in constant communication. For example, we feel nervous about a date with Ryan Gosling (or insert appropriate heartthrob). Our cardiovascular system gets involved, raising our heart rate. We feel butterflies in our stomach and we may need to rush to the bathroom. Hormones are released, such as adrenaline and cortisol, to cope with this perceived emergency. Our pupils dilate, our breath gets faster, and we freak out at what shoes we should wear. It is a full-body response to a stimulus. Therefore, it is perhaps no surprise to learn that the gut and the mind are intricately connected.

The Brain-Gut Connection

This concept is not new. In fact, in an article in *Gut Pathogens* in 2013, researchers explain that in the early 1900s, most high-profile physicians and scientists worked with the idea of "autointoxication," where the gut was viewed as the cause for any number of illnesses, particularly associated with mental health, due to the damage from unhealthy bacteria. Disturbed gut bacteria was said to contribute to fatigue, melancholia, and neuroses. Some preferred to treat drastically by suggesting the removal of part of the colon, and others suggested a manipulation of gut microbiota via the ingestion of pills and dairy-based beverages.

It's fascinating to learn that one of the first research papers written about this was in the *Journal of the American Medical Association* in 1898, which included suggestions that a lack of stomach acid may play a role in promoting undesirable microbes in the intestine, and that a change in dietary habits along with the toxins from the gut is a major contributor to depressive states. This is very similar to the view we have today. There were a number of other studies published at that time, and the concept of autointoxication was widely accepted among psychiatrists, physicians, and scientists alike.

Next came the concept that lactic acid bacteria could combat autointoxication. In 1912, the microbiologist Elie Metchnikoff wrote: "In effect, we fight microbe with microbe . . . there seems hope that we shall in time be able to transform the entire intestinal flora from a harmful to an innocuous one . . . the benefit effect of this transformation must be enormous."

Research at the time showed that *Lactobacillus bulgaricus* had a positive effect not only on mental symptoms, but also on the slowing of arteriosclerosis and other markers of age-related decline. Lactic acid bacilli tablets were made, and by 1917 an article in *Druggists Circular* (catchy name) told of about thirty different products commercially available. In the 1920s, *L. bulgaricus* was overtaken in popularity by *Lactobacillus acidophillus* as the species of choice due to its ability to live and develop in the gut. *L. acidophillus* milk was produced and sold in North America and touted almost as a cure-all. It was also during this time that research into the effect of diet on gut microbiota began emerging.

Given that there were no human trials at the time to demonstrate how this entire concept of autointoxication actually occurs, the lack of evidence caused the hypothesis to eventually run out of steam by the mid-1930s. The claims were deemed too scientifically vague. Autointoxication was said to relate only to constipation, and the idea was replaced with the view that it was the depression that caused the digestive symptoms and issues with gut flora, and not the other way around. Although the concept of autointoxication is vague and all-encompassing, it is a shame that this sort of research was not continued. Rather than being exclusively one way or the other, the answer for future research most likely lies somewhere between the two views.

It wasn't until 2003 that the notion of the connection of beneficial microbes and mental health surfaced again. The earlier reports of low stomach acid contributing to a depressed mental state have at last been backed up with more recent studies. Further research into probiotic use for mood disorders has been positive. Two separate articles in the *British Journal of Nutrition* in 2011 stated that ingestion of the *Lactobacillus helveticus* and *Bifidobacterium longum* strains led to improvements in day-to-day depression, anger, and anxiety as well as lower levels of the stress hormone cortisol.

The most recent research published in June 2013 in the journal *Gastroenterology* is the first study in humans to have found a connection running from the gut to the brain that is modulated by ingesting fermented milk. The study showed that women who consumed the fermented milk product showed engagement and communication in different parts of their brain while the group consuming no fermented milk did not.

This is a flourishing area of research, and I hope that over the coming years we will come to better understand the connection in greater detail. And there are, of course, other factors involved. Patients with mental illness show higher inflammatory markers and are more likely to experience a range of other conditions such as irritable bowel syndrome, chronic fatigue, fibromyalgia, insulin resistance, and obesity. There is also a plethora of research indicating that stress and a diet high in unhealthy fats increase the permeability of the gut lining and the development of an imbalance of bacteria.

I am very interested to follow how all of this research pans out. It is wonderful to learn more about the effect that gut bacteria has on us, and the relevance of individual strains; however, there is always a complex combination of factors involved. The fact that healthy gut bacteria and good integrity of the gut lining have a positive effect on depressive symptoms is a win for good bacteria and a win for fermenting.

Addicted to Food?

A fantastic example of the way that our food affects our gut bacteria and our mental state is found in the inability to break down large peptides from wheat and dairy. For example, in normal circumstances, once we have ingested that delicious Brie on gourmet wheat crackers, they go through two stages of digestion. First, the dairy and wheat proteins get broken down into peptides by digestive secretions released from the stomach wall. (People with suboptimal gut flora often have low stomach acid also, and so there may already be an issue at this point.) Some of these wheat and dairy peptides have chemical structures similar to the opiate morphine, and so they function in the same way in our body. They are called gluteomorphines and casomorphins. Gluteomorphines are from gliadin, a protein in gluten-containing grains such as wheat, rye, and barley. Casomorphines are from casein, the protein component of cow's milk. This process is completely normal and happens in everyone's gut.

The next stage of digestion happens in the small intestine, where the peptides are subjected to pancreatic juices on their way to the intestinal wall and are then broken down by enzymes from the microvilli of the gut cells. Each healthy gut cell (enterocyte) is armed with a smorgasbord of digestive enzymes to complete the final stage of digestion for these peptides. For those with poor gut health, this is the step where it goes awry.

Struggling gut cells are ill equipped with the enzymes to perform this task, and the gluteomorphines and casomorphins are allowed to pass into the bloodstream unchanged or improperly broken down. This causes problems not only with the immune system, as mentioned earlier, but also with brain function. Because they behave as opiates, they have sedative and addictive qualities. It looks like you may finally have an answer to why your dad falls asleep on the couch after the family lunch gathering. These two peptides can also result in irritation and inflammation in the brain, brain fog, anxiety, depression, and potentially dementia. This is why it can be so difficult for some people to stop eating bread pasta, dairy, and processed foods—it is a legitimate physiological craving. Unfortunately, the gut bacteria were not there to do their job of digesting proteins, fermenting carbohydrates, and breaking down fiber and lipids. Gut bacteria also plan an integral role in transporting vitamins and minerals, water, and other nutrients from the gut to the blood. Without healthy gut flora, the body cannot receive all the benefits from that beautiful organic broccoli. So an investment in the health of your gut and gut flora, on top of everything else you do to protect your health, is insurance that your expensive multivitamin is not going to waste!

The Link Between Gut Bacteria and Other Neurological Issues

There are many research studies illustrating that a common thread among people experiencing autism, schizophrenia, depression, and autoimmune diseases is high amounts of gluteomorphines and casomorphines in their blood. A study in the journal *Peptides* in 2009 stated that there was a relationship between high levels of casomorphins and poor psychomotor development and increased risk of autism in infants fed cow's milk.

Another study in *Expert Opinion Therapeutic Targets* in 2002 discusses the theory that opioid peptides from gluten and casein exert an effect on neurotransmission and produce a number of physiological symptoms. This study and another in *Complementary Therapies in Medicine* in 2012 found the removal of gluten and dairy to improve autistic children's behaviors and gastrointestinal symptoms. Another study, in *Peptides* in 2007, found a correlation between high levels of casomorphin and atopic dermatitis in infants who were not breast-fed.

A study in *Acta Psychiatry Scandinavia* in 2006 found a drastic reduction in schizophrenic symptoms after a gluten-free diet was introduced in a subset of schizophrenic patients. Another study, in the *Journal of Psychometric Research* in 2013, found depressive symptoms to be common among one-third of celiac disease patients, and that long-term adherence to a gluten-free diet may reduce the risk for their current depressive symptoms. A study in the *New Zealand Medical Journal* in 2012 found that a depressed mood is associated with gluten sensitivity and that a resolution of symptoms could be achieved with a gluten-free diet. And finally, a study in *Bipolar Disorder* in 2010 reported a relationship between dietary casein antigens and bipolar disorder, in that high amounts of antigens were present in those with the disorder.

So What Does All This Mean?

I've just thrown a lot of study results at you. Each one of these studies shows support for the brain-gut connection and supports the idea that the health of our gut and gut bacteria determine the way that the food we eat will be absorbed and how it will affect us both physically and emotionally.

However, it is not just about removing gluten from the diet; the gut must be repaired and bacteria restored. As an article in *Chronic Illness* in 2012 pointed out, despite adhering to a gluten-free diet, a substantial portion of their study participants still reported symptoms of depression and psychosocial distress. This highlights the fact that we need to go beyond removing the trigger in order to nourish and repair the gut. We don't have the science to know exactly what each strain of bacteria does in every situation, and so taking a formulated probiotic of specific strains may be a slightly more reductionist view. There is no doubt that we have research to vouch for the effectiveness of particular strains in alleviating certain health conditions, along with a move toward a "probiotic materia medica" whereby only certain strains are proven to be effective in a given situation rather than just being generally applied across the board. Although it is wonderful to have the research on specific strains, I believe that a holistic approach is the way forward for the general population. Fermented beverages and fermented foods have this holistic advantage of containing not only a wide range of bacteria, but also potentially other healthful substances and accompanying interactions that we do not yet know about. Fermented beverages have the ability to heal the digestive system—and they are a lot more cost-effective than purchasing probiotic supplements!

Putting It into Practice

- Supplementation with good bacteria showed an increase in hair growth and shine, an increase in skin thickness, and a general "healthful glow." Also, by improving the bacteria in our gut with fermented beverages, we encourage a more acidic environment, leading to shiny hair and radiant skin.

- Fermented milk drinks have been shown to reduce and prevent skin dryness and encourage correct skin cell replication. Certain bacteria have also been shown to produce hyaluronic acid, which assists in wound healing and tissue repair of the skin, and it also plays a role in the maintenance of skin elasticity and correct cell proliferation. Fermented beverages also contain lactic acid, a natural form of alpha hydroxy acid (AHA), which promotes collagen formation and the production of skin cells and helps reduce the signs of aging.

- The link between the gut and the brain has long been established, and recent studies show that poor digestive health and unhealthy gut bacteria are linked to a depressed mental state. Studies have shown that supplementation with healthy bacteria improves symptoms of day-to-day depression, anger, and anxiety, and lowers the levels of the stress hormone cortisol.

RECIPES AT A GLANCE

Cultured and Fermented Beverage Recipes for Radient Skin and a Healthy Mind

Blood-Cleansing Beauty Kombucha

This recipe uses fresh beet juice, which is not only delicious but also has wondrous blood-cleansing and liver-assisting properties. Full of phytonutrients, it is also a good source of iron, improving the production and nourishment of red blood cells. Because of all this, it tends to help the skin glow with good health!

1 cup (235 ml) Basic Kombucha (page 32)

1 cup (235 ml) beet juice

Mix both ingredients together and drink! If you are using freshly squeezed beet juice, this drink will tend to separate if left to sit, so enjoy right away or give it a good stir before drinking.

Yield: 2 cups (475 ml)

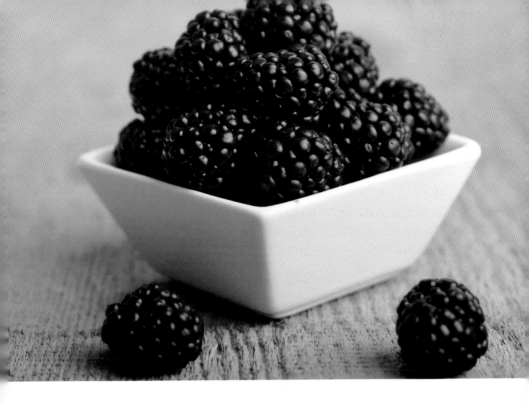

Berry Antioxidant Kombucha

This beauty contains the antioxidant benefits of green tea and acai berry powder, which is loaded with athocyanins and flavovoids, two other powerful antioxidants. Top it off with some blueberries and you have a powerful tonic to reduce oxidation and damage to the body and skin cells.

2 cups (475 ml) Basic Kombucha (page 32) made with green tea instead of black tea

¼ cup (37 g) blueberries or blackberries (preferably organic)

½ teaspoon acai berry powder

Place all of the ingredients into a glass jar and leave at room temperature to ferment for 2 days.

Strain out the berries and enjoy right away, or store in an airtight bottle in the refrigerator for up to 1 month.

Yield: 2 cups (475 ml)

Exotic Orange and Saffron Kombucha

Saffron threads are the dried stigmas of the crocus flower. Each flower contains only three stigmas, and to get 1 ounce (28 g) of saffron requires the collection of around 14,000 stigmas. It may seem expensive to buy, but because you only need a few threads in a dish, it works out as good value. Saffron is such a treat, and it is simply amazing that a few tiny strands can give such color and flavor!

2 cups (475 ml) Basic Kombucha (page 32) made with rooibos tea instead of black tea

3 (4 x 1-inch, or 10 x 2.5-cm) strips orange zest, with as little pith left on as possible

6 strands saffron

Place all of the ingredients into a glass jar and leave at room temperature to ferment for 2 days.

Strain out the orange zest and saffron and enjoy right away, or store in an airtight bottle in the refrigerator for up to 1 month.

Yield: 2 cups (475 ml)

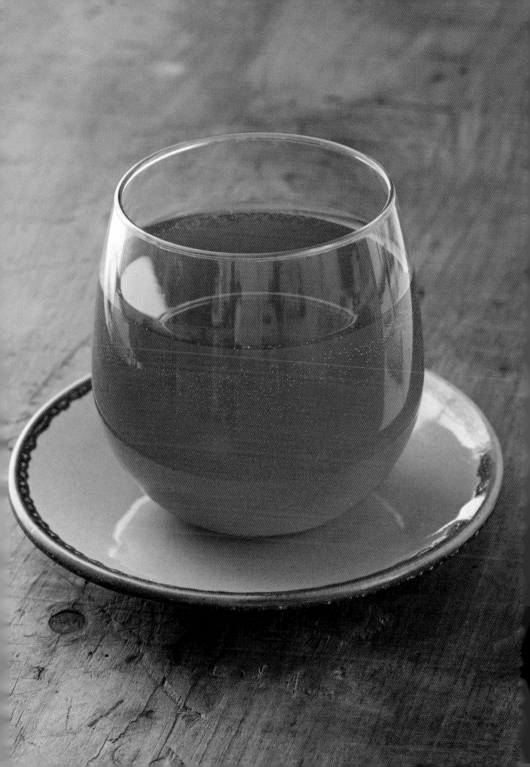

Fermented Skin-Cleansing Smoothie

Alkalizing foods are wonderful for our skin, and this cleansing drink is packed full of them, plus a load of anti-inflammatory nutrients to help reduce skin redness and irritation.

1 green apple, cored (preferably organic)

1 cup (235 ml) Basic Coconut Water Kefir (page 30)

1 cup (155 g) chopped pineapple

1 cup (135 g) chopped cucumber

1 cup (30 g) spinach leaves

½ avocado, pitted and peeled

1 tablespoon (15 ml) freshly squeezed lemon juice

1 (1-inch, or 2.5-cm) piece peeled fresh ginger

2 or 3 ice cubes

Place all of the ingredients into a blender and blend on high speed until smooth. This drink is best enjoyed right away.

Yield: 2 cups (475 ml)

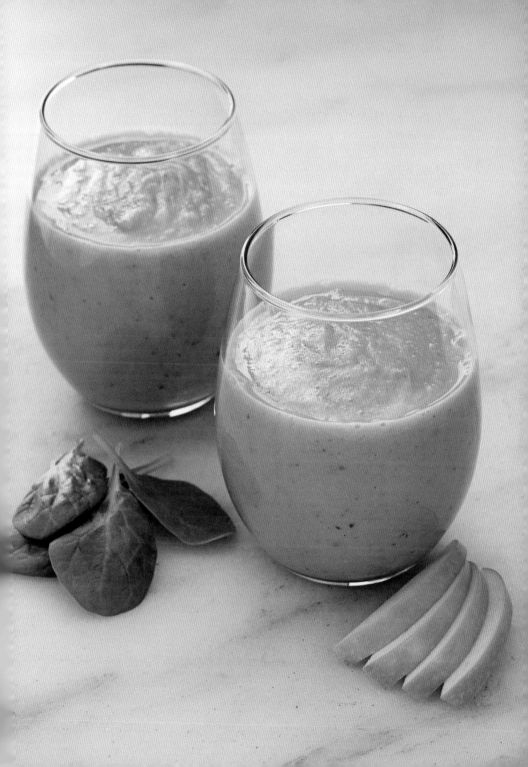

Pineapple Mint Kombucha ▸

Like a summer cocktail, this fruity number deserves a fancy glass and a little umbrella.

2 cups (475 ml) Basic Kombucha (page 32)

½ to 1 cup (80 to 155 g) chopped pineapple

1 to 2 tablespoons (6 to 12 g) fresh mint leaves

Place all of the ingredients into a blender and blend on high speed until smooth. This drink is best enjoyed right away, but will keep in an airtight bottle in the refrigerator for 1 to 2 days.

Yield: 2¼ to 2½ cups (530 to 570 ml)

White Tea, Blackberry, and Lavender Kombucha

Elegant and beautiful, this is a gorgeous floral combination. Breathe deeply and enjoy some relaxing aromatherapy from the lavender, and at the same time nourish your body with the health benefits from the kombucha and white tea. Be sure to use fresh, unsprayed food-grade lavender.

2 cups (475 ml) Basic Kombucha (page 32) made with white tea instead of black tea

¼ cup (37 g) blackberries or blueberries (preferably organic)

½ teaspoon fresh lavender blossoms

¼ teaspoon pure vanilla extract (optional)

Place all of the ingredients into a glass jar and leave at room temperature to ferment for 2 days.

Strain out the berries and lavender and enjoy right away, or store in an airtight bottle in the refrigerator for up to 1 month.

Yield: 2 cups (475 ml)

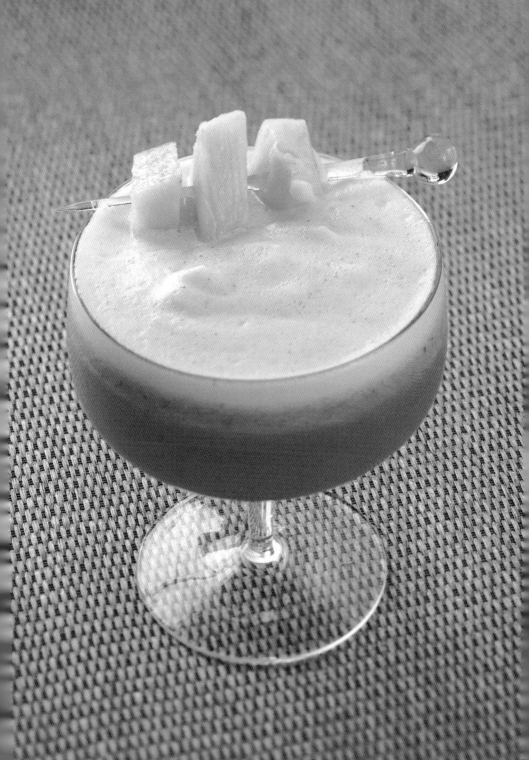

Watermelon, Lime, and Mint Kefir ▸

This is a very popular flavor combination, and with kefir included, you get not only the taste sensation but the gut goodness too!

2 cups (300 g) coarsely chopped watermelon

1 cup (235 ml) Basic Water Kefir (page 26)

1 to 2 tablespoons (15 to 30 ml) freshly squeezed lime juice

2 tablespoons (12 g) fresh mint leaves

Place the watermelon, kefir, lime juice, and half of the mint in a blender and blend on high speed until smooth. Use the rest of the mint as garnish for individual servings. Because of the fast-fermenting nature of melon, this drink is best enjoyed right away.

Yield: 2 cups (475 ml)

Brain Juice Kefir

This brew contains herbs that are high in a compound called cineole, which is a mild stimulant, providing a nice little pick-me-up without the caffeine jitters that normally come with other energy drinks. Squeeze a bit of lemon juice into the drink before serving, if you like.

2 cups (475 ml) Basic Water Kefir (page 26)

6 to 8 fresh mint leaves

4 fresh sage leaves

2 bay leaves

Sprig of fresh rosemary

½ teaspoon ground turmeric or 1 teaspoon grated fresh turmeric

Place all of the ingredients into a glass jar and leave at room temperature to ferment for 2 days.

Strain out the berries and enjoy right away, or store in an airtight bottle in the refrigerator for up to 1 month.

Yield: 2 cups (475 ml)

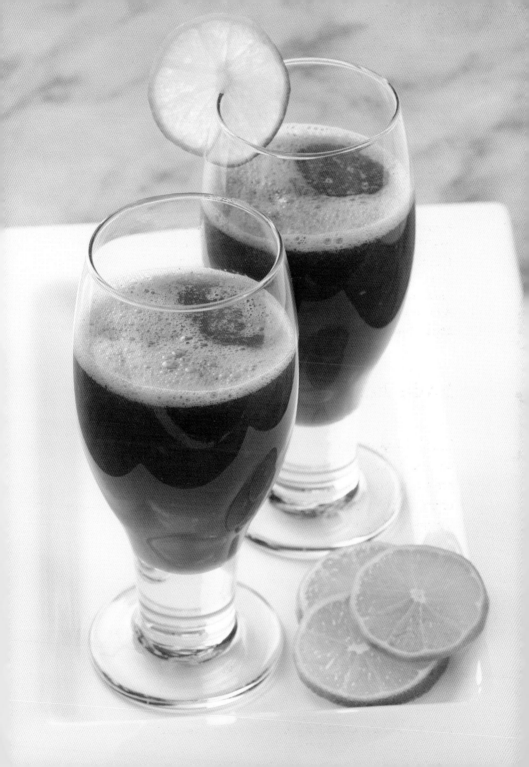

Pomegranate Kefir Cocktail

This zesty cocktail is lovely on its own, and it makes a great base for a vodka cocktail. I'm just saying.

1 cup (235 ml) Basic Water Kefir (page 26) or Basic Coconut Water Kefir (page 30)

½ cup (120 ml) pomegranate juice

¼ cup (60 ml) freshly squeezed orange juice

1 to 2 teaspoons freshly squeezed lemon or lime juice

Ice cubes (optional)

Combine all of the ingredients in a large glass and enjoy right away.

Yield: 1¾ cups (425 ml)

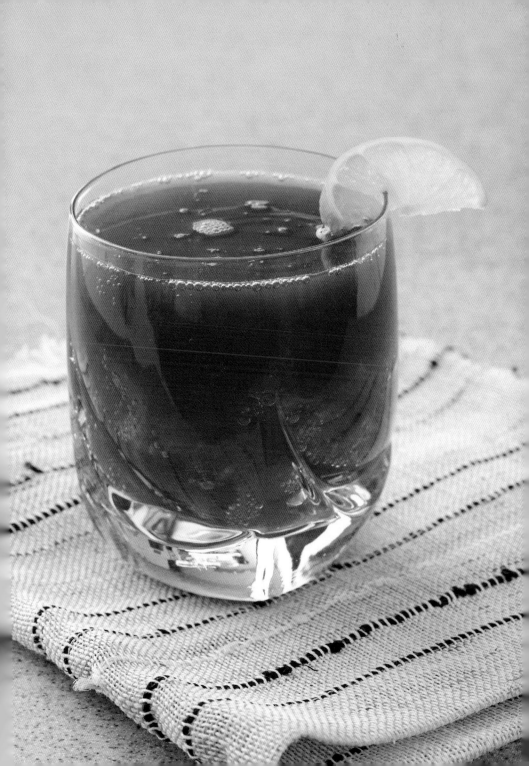

Gorgeous Green Basil, Mango, and Passion Fruit Kefir

The addition of the kefir to these wonderful fruits and veg makes for a serious health beverage. The passion fruit can be whizzed up in the smoothie together with the rest of the ingredients, or sprinkled on top as directed.

1 ripe mango, peeled, pitted, and chopped

1 cup (67 g) chopped kale

8 to 10 fresh basil leaves

1½ cups (355 ml) Basic Water Kefir (page 26) or Basic Coconut Water Kefir (page 30)

1½ teaspoons freshly squeezed lemon juice

1 passion fruit, seeds and pulp coarsely chopped

Place the mango, kale, basil, kefir, and lemon juice into a blender and blend on high speed until smooth. Serve in glasses sprinkled with the passion fruit seeds and pulp.

Yield: 2 cups (475 ml)

Pomegranate Apple Soda

You can ferment absolutely any flavorings you like to make a cultured soda. This combination of apple and pomegranate is refreshing and delicious.

½ cup (120 ml) water, plus more to fill up the bottles

¼ to ¾ cup (50 to 150 g) organic white cane sugar, depending on taste

1 pound (455 g) apples, cored and coarsely chopped (preferably organic)

¼ cup (50 g) pomegranate arils (or pomegranate juice if you prefer)

¼ cup ginger bug or turmeric syrup (page 119)

3 tablespoons (45 ml) freshly squeezed lemon juice

Bring the ½ cup (120 ml) water to a boil in a large saucepan. Add the sugar, stirring until dissolved. Stir in the apples, take the mixture off the heat, and allow to cool completely.

Transfer the mixture to a blender and blend on high speed until smooth.

Push the mixture through a fine-mesh strainer or a nut milk bag to drain as much of the syrupy juice as you can into a small bowl.

Pour the juice into a 1-liter bottle and add water to fill the bottle about two-thirds full. Add the pomegranate arils, ginger bug, and lemon juice, making sure there is still about 1 inch (2.5 cm) of space left at the top.

Allow to sit at room temperature covered with a piece of cheesecloth. Once your mixture begins to bubble vigorously (this may take a day or a few days depending on the room temperature), it is time to cap it and let it sit in a dark place for at least another 2 days to carbonate. Keep checking on your soda, because if you let the carbonation build up too much, your bottle will explode. Burp your bottle frequently by loosening the lid and allowing the air to escape, and then replace the lid.

Once you have reached the carbonation level that you are happy with, drink it, or transfer to the refrigerator to slow down the fermenting process.

Yield: 4¼ cups (1 liter)

CHAPTER 6

Botanical Fermentation: Cultured Herbs for Basic Health Conditions

Herbal medicine harks back to prehistoric times, and it is still the most widely used form of health care in the world today. In fact, the World Health Organization estimates that around 80 percent of people living in some countries throughout Asia and Africa use herbal medicine as their primary source of health care. Traditional doctors in ancient times collected and collated information about herbs over thousands of years, and now we have the benefit of scientific studies to enlighten us further about these precious medicines. Plants have wonderful abilities to perform myriad helpful functions within the body.

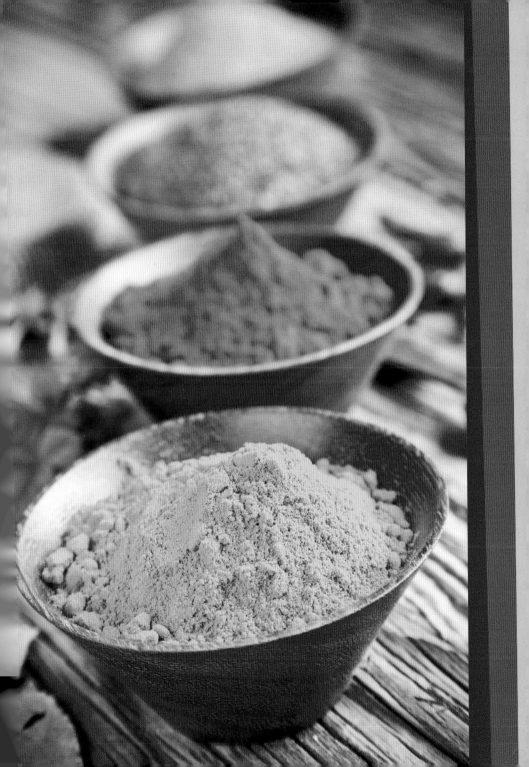

Modern pharmaceutical medicine has a lot to thank herbal medicine for, given that many drugs are derived from herbs or plants. The most common example is the willow tree, whose bark contains salicylic acid—the active metabolite of aspirin. Also digoxin, the heart drug, is derived from the plant foxglove.

The wonderful thing about herbal medicine is that it often presents fewer side effects for the user than chemical medicine, as it generally works with the body to achieve a goal rather than overriding your own healing ability.

According to the American Botanical Council, top-selling herbal remedies in the United States include cranberry, saw palmetto, garlic, ginkgo, echinacea, milk thistle, black cohosh, St. John's wort, and ginseng. They address issues including urinary tract infections, prostate health, immunity support, liver support, hormonal balance, mood lifting, and energy promotion. These top herbs cover a wide range of conditions and illustrate the scope of herbal medicine.

Herbal extracts can be prepared a number of ways. The two main methods for commercial use include maceration and percolation. With maceration, herbs are steeped in a solvent at room temperature for 1 to 2 weeks. In percolation, the solvent slowly drips through a tall vessel containing the herbs.

In addition to these methods, there is also decoction (simmering the herb for about half an hour), infusion (steeping the plant material in water, as you would make a cup of tea), and expression (extracting the juice by pulping and pressing the herb).

Although scarce, there are a number of exciting studies emerging showing the process of fermenting herbs to have a beneficial effect on the herbs' properties and constituents. One study from the *Journal of Ethnopharmacology* in 2012 found that fermented ginseng, when compared with nonfermented ginseng, produced fifteen times more of a particular metabolite that has antitumor effects. In 2012 research in *Bioscience, Biotechnology and Biochemistry* found fermented green tea to reduce the effect of alcohol-induced liver damage.

A study in the *Journal of Herbal Medicine and Toxicology* in 2010 researched the effect of fermentation on *Phyllanthis niruri*, a traditional Ayurvedic herb known to have an antimicrobial effect. The herb was fermented two ways: first using the natural Lactobacillus found on the herb surface, and second using a commercial strain of *Lactobacillus acidophilus*. The results showed that the antimicrobial potential of the herb increased by 80 to 170 percent when compared to the crude extract. Furthermore, the researchers found that the herb fermented using the Lactobacillus from the herb's surface was 49 percent more potent than when using the commercial *Lactobacillus acidophilus* isolates. Another study, in *Phytotherapy Research* in 2009, demonstrated increased bioavailability and immunity modulating ability of various fermented herbs in relation to the treatment of atopic dermatitis. Although there is not an abundance of information in this area, the studies that have been done are very promising, and it makes for a wonderful new area of research.

It is fascinating to apply this principle to any herb that you may choose to ferment, in that it is possible that fermenting may improve the potency or healthful qualities. We don't know how fermenting chamomile, for example, would change its qualities, but it is exciting to consider that it may increase the herb's effectiveness. It is also a good time to point out that as we don't know exactly what constituents of the herbs are changed by fermentation, care must be taken if taking any prescription medication or if there is any chronic illness. Check with your health care practitioner about the appropriateness of particular herbs for you.

Herbal Assistance for Common Health Issues

Following are some useful herbs and spices to help treat common health complaints. I have listed their main actions, but please take note that if you have a chronic health condition, or if you are pregnant or breast-feeding, you should consult your health care practitioner before fermenting these herbs. The list that follows is by no means exhaustive, and the recipes that follow in this chapter do not use every one of them, but I believe that these herbs would work well with the fermentation process as a second ferment. So please do experiment!

For healing the gut and promoting digestive health, we already know how great fermented beverages are on their own. For more specific complaints, adding herbs to the mix can give ferments a whole new perspective.

DANDELION

Dandelion is one of my favorite herbs. It is an effective digestive stimulant, it assists with reducing bloating, and it is amazing for the liver.

CHAMOMILE

Chamomile is like a big hug for your tummy! It is a carminitive, so it relaxes your intestinal muscles to relieve pain or cramping. It is wonderful for that feeling of trapped gas, and it helps reduce flatulence and can assist the alleviating symptoms of irritable bowel syndrome (IBS). Chamomile is anti-inflammatory and also a mild nervous system relaxant, helping to reduce anxiety. It is a wonderful remedy for children, particularly those who experience colic or hyperactivity.

FENNEL

Fennel is not only delicious but is also an effective herb for calming the digestive system. Similar to chamomile, it is a carminitive, so it decreases bloating and flatulence as it directs warming energy to your gut. In this way, it can help in situations where the digestive fire is weak. Traditionally, it has been used for colic as well.

PEPPERMINT

Perhaps best known for reducing nausea, peppermint is a carminitive and reduces spasm and pain in the digestive tract. It is also helpful in reducing gas and bloating.

TURMERIC

Anti-inflammatory, antioxidant, antimicrobial, carminitive, and cholesterol reducing, turmeric is a superhero, and I can only imagine what fermenting it might do for its potential!

GINGER

Another anti-inflammatory heavyweight, ginger plays a role in assisting digestion, reducing pain, and relieving nausea—especially morning sickness—and is antimicrobial. It is a warming herb that assists circulation and brings energy to the digestive system.

CINNAMON

Cinnamon is another warming herb that is useful for digestive complaints such as loss of appetite, diarrhea, mild cramping, and gas. Cinnamon also has some lovely research supporting its use for diabetes in terms of increased insulin sensitivity. It's also antibacterial and antifungal.

Given that 80 percent of our immune system resides in our gut, the two are inextricably connected. Fermented beverages alone will work to improve general immunity; however, there are some wonderful herbs that can give you a further boost.

ECHINACEA

Echinacea is one of the most well-known herbs for the immune system. On top of its immunostimulant and immunomodulatory actions, it is a lymphatic, which means that it improves the flow of lymph and the detoxification of the body. It is most useful in treating upper respiratory infections and enhancing the immune response of the body.

CALENDULA

Calendula is a lymphatic and anti-inflammatory, often used in any inflammation of the throat or mouth but also for inflamed lymph nodes, ulcers, cysts, and some reproductive conditions. Topically, it encourages the healing of wounds.

ELDERFLOWER

Elderflower is a beautiful herb for the common cold or flu. It assists in clearing out phlegm and also encourages sweating to control a fever. It can be useful in treating sinusitis, hay fever, sore throat, and bronchitis.

SAGE

Because of its astringent, antioxidant, and antimicrobial nature, sage is perfect for sore throats or any infection or inflammation in the mouth or throat. It can also be useful in alleviating excessive sweating, hot flashes, and night sweating, but keep away if you're breast-feeding, as sage is traditionally used to stop milk flow. It is also not suitable for use during pregnancy.

GARLIC

Ever since garlic was discovered—and what a great day that was—it has been used as food and as medicine. The ancient Egyptians used it to ward off infection, Sanskrit records note the use of garlic dating back 5,000 years, and it was used in both world wars to prevent gangrene and treat infection. It is a fabulous herb for treating and preventing colds, flu, and coughs due to its antimicrobial and immune-enhancing acidity. The catch with garlic is that the active constituent allicin works best when unheated. So fermenting is perfect!

THYME

Another fabulous herb for sore throats, thyme is antibacterial, antifungal, antimicrobial, and antioxidant. It's also wonderful for treating coughs or any congestion of the upper respiratory tract.

The addition of the following herbs to your fermented brews will give them a different dimension. Whether it's relaxation, adrenal support, or a little help with sleep that you are after, one of the following herbs should set you on the right path.

LICORICE

Licorice is one of my favorite herbs. It is a wonderful adrenal tonic, supporting and improving the function of our adrenal glands, which get a bashing during times of prolonged stress. Aside from the nervous system, licorice has a role to play in the treatment of coughs, gastric ulcers or reflux, and some reproductive conditions. If taking any potassium-depleting drugs such as thiazide, diuretics, or laxatives, the prolonged intake of licorice may add to the further loss of potassium and should be monitored.

PASSIONFLOWER

A beautiful herb—even the name is gorgeous! Passionflower relieves anxiety, nervous tension, restlessness, and irritability. It also assists with sleep and the symptoms of anxiety, including a racing heart rate or headaches. It is mildly sedating.

LAVENDER

Lavender is well known for its relaxing aromatherapy benefits, and taken internally it has a similar effect. Restlessness, anxiety, low mood, and insomnia are all conditions in which lavender is helpful. Lavender would be best used in a second ferment due to its natural oil content.

VALERIAN

Valerian is not only a sleep-inducing herb, but it is also used to help decrease states of stress and anxiety.

LEMON BALM

This is one herb for which I did find some research regarding fermenting. A study in *Romanian Biotechnological Letters* from 2013 showed lemon balm to be a good substitute for black tea as a medium for kombucha SCOBYs, and that the length of time taken to ferment was less than that of the traditional black tea. The study compared lemon balm, peppermint, thyme, and sage, with peppermint and thyme coming out as second and third best, and sage not recommended due to the length of time taken to ferment.

Lemon balm is a gentle herb used to help with sleep, nervous tension, and irritability. There is a lovely crossover with the gut, and for those who feel their nervousness in the gut, this is a wonderful herb to choose. Carrying on the gut qualities, lemon balm may also ease indigestion, gas, and colic.

Other Useful Herbs and Plants

Although not technically part of the "herbal medicine" family, the following plants can be used in a similar manner. They have many health-giving qualities and work beautifully as a base for fermenting.

Green tea is not technically an herb, but rather is from the same plant, *Camellia sinensis*, as black tea; it involves a different processing technique. Black tea is rolled and fermented, whereas green tea is steamed first to prevent any initial fermentation. Green tea has a long list of health benefits. It contains catechins, which are a type of antioxidant that have a powerful effect on the body. A particular catechin, epigallocatechin-3-gallate (EGCG), is associated with being anticancer, antiobesity, antiatherosclerotic, antidiabetic, antibacterial, and antiviral; it can reduce dental cavities.

Green tea is anticarcinogenic in a number of ways. It assists in the process of detoxifying carcinogens from the diet by increasing phase II liver detoxification and reducing the formation of reactive and damaging intermediates from phase I detoxification. A study in *Nature Reviews Cancer* in 2009 shows that green tea also interferes with the proliferation of cancer cells, encourages correct cell signaling, inhibits cell invasion, and limits metastasis (the spread of cancer to other parts of the body). Research published in the journal *Chinese Medicine* in 2008 shows the greatest effectiveness with breast cancer and ovarian cancer. On top of this, it encourages the process of programmed cell death called apoptosis. Basically, this process is like quality control, making sure everything is running smoothly and improving the quality of workmanship.

In relation to obesity-related insulin resistance, a study in *BMC Pharmacology* in 2004 showed green tea to improve insulin sensitivity. The consumption of green tea is associated with a reduced risk of type 2 diabetes via its effect of reducing fasting blood glucose levels by regulating liver enzymes.

Green tea may contribute to a reduction in body weight and fat by increasing energy expenditure and promoting the utilization of fat (*Journal of Nutritional Biochemistry*, 2011). An article in *Molecular Nutrition and Food Research* in 2012 suggests that this is due to EGCG's ability to stimulate the liver's metabolism of fat, and also via the inhibition of the production of fat via lipogenesis (the process by which glucose is converted into fatty acids).

Other components of green tea, theaninine and aminobutyric acid, are known to lower blood pressure and regulate brain and nerve function. Green tea also contains vitamin C for better immune function and extra antioxidant activity.

So what happens when you ferment it? A study in *Bioscience Biotechnology and Biochemistry* in 2012 showed green tea that was fermented with the *Lactobacilli fermentum* strain reduced the risk of alcohol-induced liver damage. It does this by increasing the level of alcohol dehydrogenase, an enzyme that is responsible for metabolizing alcohol into acetaldehyde and then to harmless acetic acid.

Yerba maté is an herbal tea infusion made from the leaves of the *Ilex paraguariensis* tree. It is widely consumed in South America. A study from the *Comprehensive*

Reviews in Food Science Technology and Food Safety in 2010 states that it has the largest antioxidant and polyphenol content among all tea-based and non-tea-based drinks. Yerba maté does have caffeine, and also theobromine, alkaloids, flavonoids, amino acids, minerals, and vitamins C, B_1, and B_2.

Chemically a great substitute for black tea when brewing kombucha, yerba maté has been shown to display health benefits of its own. A study in the *Journal of Food Science* in 2007, and another in the *Journal of Ethnopharmacology* in 2011, lists several positive effects, including lowering cholesterol, protecting the liver, antioxidant properties, various cardiovascular benefits, and protecting against cigarette-induced lung inflammation.

Although yerba maté contains caffeine, the benefits and nutritional profile help counteract the typical caffeine side effects of nervousness or a post-energy crash.

Rooibos (pronounced ROY-bos) is a fermented herbal tea made from the South African shrub *Aspalathus linearis*. It is caffeine-free and has very little tannins, so it tastes naturally quite sweet. It is high in antioxidants, particularly polyphenols, including aspalathin, nothofagin, quercetin, rutin, and luteolin. Catchy names perhaps not, but they play an integral role in reducing vascular inflammation, which is a contributing factor to heart disease and stroke. Rooibos tea contains minerals such as potassium, copper, calcium, zinc, manganese, and magnesium, and it also increases iron absorption.

Rooibos has also been shown to be antimutagenic, anti-inflammatory, hypoglycemic, cardioprotective, and modulating of oxidative stress.

Putting It into Practice

- Herbal medicine often presents fewer side effects than pharmaceutical drugs, and it is designed to work with the body to achieve a particular goal rather than overriding the body's potential.

- Some studies are emerging that show that fermenting herbs may have a positive effect on the herb's properties and constituents. Research has demonstrated increased bioavailability of various fermented herbs as compared to the raw herbs. It is exciting to consider the potential for fermentation of herbs.

- Because there are few studies and little information on fermenting herbs, you have a wonderful opportunity to experiment, using the following recipes as a jumping-off point. Of course, if you are pregnant, breast-feeding, or have any health condition, please consult your health care practitioner before doing so.

Cultured and Fermented Beverage Recipes Featuring Healthful Herbs and Spices

Morning Boost Kombucha

Maca is a traditional root plant native to mountainous areas of Peru. It is rich in calcium, magnesium, phosphorous, potassium, iron, and B vitamins and has a wonderful antioxidant profile. Traditionally, maca has been used to improve physical endurance and enhance both cognitive and sexual function. It is also said to balance the endocrine system via its promotion of optimal functioning of the hypothalamus and pituitary glands. This recipe includes maca but also ginger and cayenne to really kick the metabolism and circulation into action.

2 cups (475 ml) Basic Kombucha (page 32)

10 slices fresh ginger (do not peel)

1 teaspoon maca powder

⅛ to ¼ teaspoon cayenne pepper

Place all of the ingredients into a glass jar and put on the lid. Leave the bottle out of direct sunlight at room temperature for 2 days.

Strain out the ginger and store in an airtight bottle in the refrigerator for up to 1 month.

Yield: 2 cups (475 ml)

Digestive Tonic

The combination of these three herbs helps reduce pain and bloating in the digestive tract. The chamomile and lemon balm also have a calming effect on the nervous system. Rooibos is used for the base kombucha tea to keep caffeine out of the equation. This is the perfect after-dinner tea.

2 cups (475 ml) Basic Kombucha (page 32) made with rooibos tea instead of black tea

1 teaspoon dried chamomile flowers

1 teaspoon dried lemon balm

1 teaspoon dried peppermint

Place all of the ingredients into a glass jar and put on the lid. Leave the bottle out of direct sunlight at room temperature for 2 days.

Strain out the herbs and store in an airtight bottle in the refrigerator for up to 1 month.

Yield: 2 cups (475 ml)

Kefir Gut Healer

Slippery elm powder is the ground inner bark of the slippery elm tree. It is hydrophilic, meaning it is able to trap water within and then swells and becomes gelatinous. Once consumed, it is broken down by the gut bacteria and has a soothing effect on gastrointestinal inflammation and irritation and helps alleviate symptoms of conditions such as diarrhea, gastritis, reflux, peptic ulcers, and irritable bowel syndrome. Slippery elm powder also contains vitamin C, zinc, magnesium, ion, potassium, and B vitamins. The catch? It is not the most palatable thing in the world. Slippery elm powder is most likely not your typical addition to your daily beverage, but it combines nicely in this drink. It makes friends well with the banana, cacao, and cinnamon, and the turmeric is there to play its own role as a major anti-inflammatory spice that's beneficial for the gut. Feel free to play around with the quantities to find a ratio that works for you.

1 cup (235 ml) Basic Coconut Milk Kefir (page 28) or Basic Milk Kefir (page 24) or Basic Coconut Water Kefir (page 30)

½ banana

1 to 2 teaspoons slippery elm powder (start with 1)

1 teaspoon raw cacao powder

¼ teaspoon ground cinnamon

¼ teaspoon ground turmeric

Place all of the ingredients into a blender and blend until smooth. Enjoy right away. Left unattended, the slippery elm will absorb a lot of the liquid, and you will end up with quite a thick pudding.

Yield: 1 cup (235 ml)

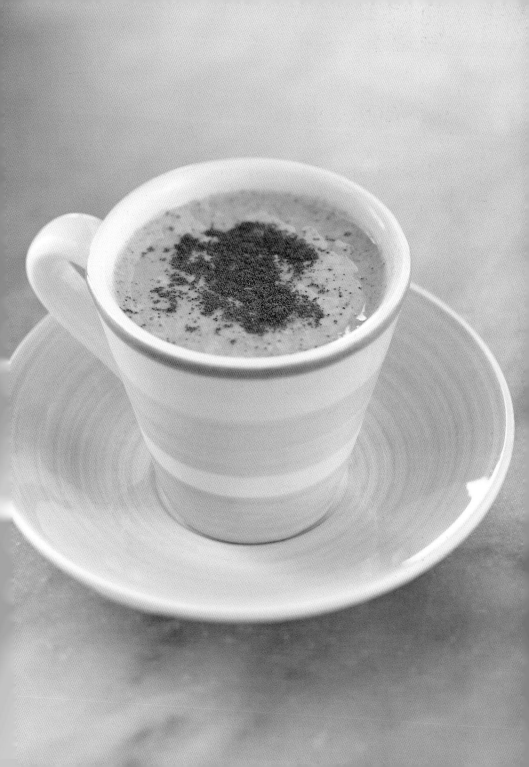

Stress Less Kombucha

This combination of lemon balm and licorice is not only delicious, but it will also help relax both your digestive and your nervous systems. Lemon balm is the perfect herb for those who feel their anxiety in their guts, and licorice is nourishing and healing to the adrenal glands.

2 cups (475 ml) water

¼ cup (50 g) organic white or rapadura (panela) sugar

1 tablespoon (2 g) dried lemon balm

1 kombucha SCOBY

½ cup (120 ml) Basic Kombucha (page 32)

½ to 1 teaspoon cut and sifted licorice root

In a saucepan, bring the water to a boil, then add the sugar, stirring to dissolve. Add the lemon balm to the water (or use a tea ball), and leave to cool completely.

Strain out the tea leaves, and transfer the cooled tea to a wide-mouth jar. Add the SCOBY and kombucha, and leave to ferment according to the Basic Kombucha recipe on page 32.

Once finished, transfer 2 cups of the kombucha to a jar with the licorice root. Put a lid on the jar and leave to ferment for 1 day.

Strain out the licorice, and store the kombucha in an airtight bottle in the refrigerator for up to 1 month.

Yield: 2 cups (475 ml)

Dandelion Tea Smoothie

Dandelion tea is best known for its effect on the liver, assisting it in the production of bile. It is also a bitter tonic for the digestive system, helping to stimulate digestive secretions.

1 cup (235 ml) water

1 dandelion root tea bag

½ cup (120 ml) Basic Milk Kefir (page 24)

½ to 1 banana

½ teaspoon ground cinnamon

In a saucepan, bring the water to a boil. Add the tea bag and steep for 5 minutes.

Add the brewed tea and all of the remaining ingredients to a blender and blend on high speed until smooth. Enjoy right away.

Yield: 1½ cups (355 ml)

Morning Glorious

When visiting my lovely friend Suzie one day, we had lunch at a café where I tasted an amazing chocolate-coffee smoothie. Nothing fermented, but it was delicious, and I knew I wanted to make my own version of it for this book. So here it is! Although it's not technically an herb, I have included coffee in this section.

1 cup (235 ml) cultured almond coconut milk (page 104) or Basic Milk Kefir (page 24)

1 cup (235 ml) almond, oat, or rice milk, or milk of your choice

¼ cup brewed coffee, or to taste

1 banana

2 teaspoons raw cacao powder

1 to 2 teaspoons pure maple syrup, to taste

Place all of the ingredients into a blender and blend on high speed until smooth. Taste and add additional coffee or maple syrup as desired. Enjoy right away.

Yield: 2 cups (475 ml)

Post-Workout Electrolyte-Balancing Kefir

This combination has coconut water kefir for electrolytes, almonds and chia for protein, and kale and berries for added nutrients and deliciousness.

1½ cups (355 ml) Basic Coconut Water Kefir (page 30)

1 frozen banana

1 cup (145 g) blueberries or any other berry (preferably organic)

½ cup (34 g) kale or spinach leaves

¼ cup (35 g) raw unsalted almonds

2 tablespoons (25 g) chia seeds

Place all of the ingredients into a blender and blend on high speed until smooth. Enjoy right away.

Yield: 2 cups (475 ml)

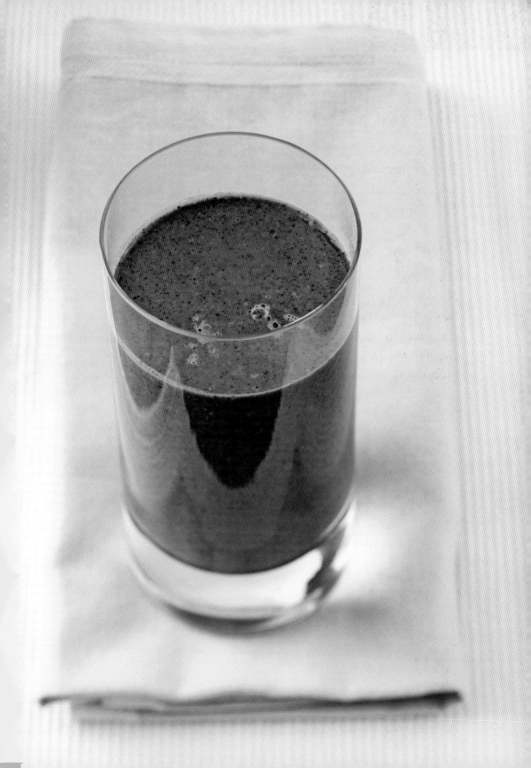

Sage and Lemon Throat Soother

Sage is antibacterial and soothing for the throat. Lemon is astringent and contains loads of vitamin C. The addition of manuka honey, which is naturally antibacterial and soothing to the throat, makes this a winner for when you are feeling under the weather.

Fresh thyme and garlic are other great optional add-ins. The thyme should not be used for fermenting, as its volatile oils may harm the bacteria, but you could add it before drinking. Also, half a chopped clove of garlic (added for its antibacterial nature) will give you an entirely different perspective.

1 cup (235 ml) Basic Water Kefir (page 26)

12 to 14 fresh sage leaves

2 slices lemon (preferably organic)

Manuka honey or other good-quality raw honey, for serving

Place the kefir, sage, and lemon slices into a glass jar, put the lid on, and leave at room temperature to ferment for 1 day, or longer if your throat can wait!

Serve with a little manuka honey, and sip small amounts as needed.

Yield: 1 cup (235 ml)

Yerba Maté Lemon Slushie

This takes me back to being a teenager, when, I am horrified to admit, I used to drink very large cups of the unfermented full-o-sugar variety. This is a tangy, icy drink that will melt quite quickly, so enjoy it fast!

2 cups (475 ml) Basic Kombucha (page 32) made with yerba maté instead of black tea (stop the fermenting before it gets too sour)

2 tablespoons (30 ml) freshly squeezed lemon juice

½ teaspoon lemon zest, or to taste

Combine all of the ingredients in a shallow freezer-safe dish and freeze for a couple of hours.

Remove from the freezer, and rake a fork over the surface firmly until you scratch up the icy mix into a slushy texture.

Transfer to glasses and enjoy pronto!

Yield: 2 cups (475 ml)

Cleansing Calendula Kombucha

Calendula is a wonderful cleansing herb, particularly for the lymphatic system. You may find that drinking this brings on small breakouts to begin with, as the skin releases toxins, but continuing on with it usually brings a radiant complexion.

2 cups (475 ml) Basic Kombucha (page 32)

2 teaspoons (1.3 g) dried calendula flowers

Place both ingredients into a glass jar, add the lid, and leave to ferment at room temperature for 2 days. Store in an airtight bottle in the refrigerator for up to 1 month.

Yield: 2 cups (475 ml)

Traditional Honey Mead

Mead is a sweet wine that is essentially fermented honey. It was traditionally used as a source of nutrients, in particular B vitamins, as well as other medicinal components. You must use raw honey for this recipe, as that is the source of the yeasts needed to culture the beverage. If the honey is pasteurized, the yeasts are killed off. According to Sandor Katz in *The Art of Fermentation*, the yeasts normally sit inactive in the honey, but once diluted with water, they revive and come to life. Other ways to make mead include adding a starter yeast to the brew, but I have chosen Sandor Katz's au naturel version.

1 cup plus 1 tablespoon (360 g) raw honey

3⅓ cups (800 ml) cold water

Dissolve the honey in the water. You may need to be patient with this, as you can imagine it takes a little persistence to dissolve honey in cold water. It is important, however, as this is the source of your yeasts to start the fermentation. You can either do this in a jar with a lid, or in a bowl. If using a jar, shake vigorously and persistently. If using a bowl, stir rapidly in one direction, and then change the direction and pull the whirlpool the opposite way.

Once dissolved, stir or shake the mead vigorously 4 or 5 times daily. After a few days, you should notice a release of bubbles as you do this. This is the yeast waking up!

This vigorous bubbling routine should continue, and after 7 to 10 days the bubbling will begin to die down. (This may take a lot longer in cold temperatures.)

The fermentation process will continue for years if you allow it; however, you can drink your mead "young" once this rapid bubbling peaks and slows. Sandor Katz explains that because honey contains both glucose and fructose, it is the glucose that initiates this rapid initial fermentation, and the fructose fermentation takes place over months. Drinking it young is traditionally how people have enjoyed their mead.

Yield: 4¼ cups (1 liter)

Wild-Crafted Dandelion Nettle Mead

This one will make you feel like a real herbalist. Go foraging for some dandelion flowers; stay away from flowers next to the roadside, as these will be quite polluted. You can take your time collecting them if you need to and freeze them in a freezer bag until you have enough. The nettle you can also forage, or you can often find it at farmers' markets depending on the time of year. Dandelion and nettle will certainly boost the liver-loving properties, and the mineral richness, of your mead.

3⅓ cups (800 ml) water

About 1 cup (30 g) dandelion flowers (snip the yellow heads off close to the top)

½ cup (15 g) nettle leaves

1 cup plus 1 tablespoon (360 g) raw honey

Bring the water to a boil. Place the dandelion and nettle in a bowl and cover with the boiling water. Once cooled, strain out the flowers and leaves and add the honey.

Once the honey is dissolved, stir or shake the mead vigorously 4 or 5 times daily. After a few days, you should notice a release of bubbles as you do this. This is the yeast waking up. This vigorous bubbling routine should continue, and after 7 to 10 days the bubbling will begin to die down. (This may take a lot longer in cold temperatures.)

The fermentation process will continue for years if you allow it; however, you can drink your mead "young" once this rapid bubbling peaks and slows. Sandor Katz explains that because honey contains both glucose and fructose, it is the glucose that initiates this rapid initial fermentation, and the fructose fermentation takes place over months. Drinking it young is traditionally how people have enjoyed their mead.

Yield: 4¼ cups (1 liter)

Chamomile Vanilla Mead

I love this combination of chamomile and vanilla with the sweet honey of the mead. A wonderful after-dinner drink, this beverage is soothing and relaxing for both the gut and the nervous system.

3⅓ cups (800 ml) water

1 cup (25 g) dried chamomile flowers

1 cup plus 1 tablespoon (360 g) raw honey

1 vanilla bean, split

Bring the water to a boil. Place the chamomile flowers in a bowl and cover with the boiling water. Once cooled completely, strain out the chamomile, add the honey, and stir to combine. Transfer to a bottle and add the vanilla bean.

Stir or shake the mead vigorously 4 or 5 times daily. After a few days, you should notice a release of bubbles as you do this. This is the yeast waking up. This vigorous bubbling routine should continue, and after 7 to 10 days the bubbling will begin to die down. (This may take a lot longer in cold temperatures.)

The fermentation process will continue for years if you allow it; however, you can drink your mead "young" once this rapid bubbling peaks and slows. Sandor Katz explains that because honey contains both glucose and fructose, it is the glucose that initiates this rapid initial fermentation, and the fructose fermentation takes place over months. Drinking it young is traditionally how people have enjoyed their mead.

Yield: 4¼ cups (1 liter)

Lacto-Fermented Elderflower Soda

This soda uses a different starter: whey. Whey is the watery liquid that forms on the top of yogurt once it's been in the refrigerator. See the simple recipe that follows for how to make your own whey.

4¼ cups (1 liter) water

¼ to ½ cup (7 to 13 g) dried elderflowers

2 tablespoons (40 g) raw honey

¾ cup (175 ml) whey (recipe follows)

2 slices fresh ginger or turmeric (unpeeled)

Whey (plus Bonus Cream Cheese)

1½ cups (345 g) full-fat plain yogurt or (355 ml) Basic Milk Kefir (page 24)

Place a piece of cheesecloth or a thin, lint-free kitchen towel over a small bowl. Place the yogurt or kefir into the middle of the cloth, gather the sides together, and secure at the top with an elastic band or piece of string. Hang the cloth on a hook or cupboard handle above the bowl and allow to drip into the bowl overnight.

In the morning, you will have a bowl full of pale-colored liquid—this is the whey. Transfer to an airtight bottle and store in the refrigerator for up to 6 months. The yogurt or kefir left in the cloth is now cream cheese, and this will keep for a least a couple of weeks, or longer, stored in the refrigerator.

Makes about ¾ cup (175 ml)

Bring the water to a boil. Place the elderflowers in a bowl and cover with the boiling water. Allow to cool completely, and then strain out the flowers. Add the honey.

Place the whey into a 1-liter jar and top up with the elderflower infusion until 2 inches (5 cm) below the top. Add the ginger or turmeric. Cover with cheesecloth and leave to sit at room temperature out of sunlight for 2 to 3 days.

Enjoy right away, or store in an airtight bottle in the refrigerator for up to 1 month. Keep checking, as your soda will continue to slowly ferment, and you may need to release the air pressure every now and then.

Yield: 4¼ cups (1 liter)

CHAPTER 7

Tools of the Trade and Frequently Asked Questions

It was important to me to have these recipes be easy and simple to make at home, with no fancy equipment or complicated procedures. I also kept the yield sizes small for this reason, but you should feel free to double and triple recipes.

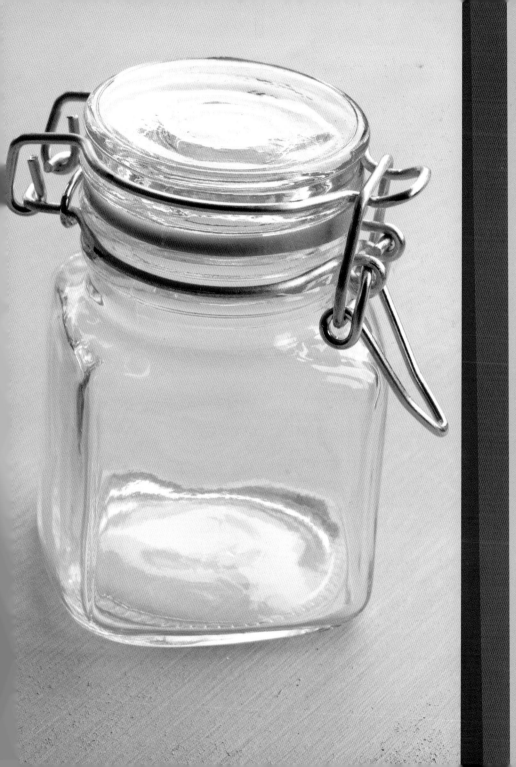

TOOLS

There is nothing out of the ordinary in the following equipment list; there are no fancy, hard-to-find items or giant contraptions that will take over your kitchen. I have purposely kept it small scale to show how easily fermented beverages can be incorporated into your kitchen and your life.

A Collection of Mixing Bowls

You will need at least one glass or ceramic bowl to make any of the ferments. I find that I use a 4-cup (946-ml) capacity one the most for the batches of kombucha or kefir that I make.

Canning Jars and Fermenting Vessels

I have a thing with collecting jars. I love to keep everything in them: nuts, grains, smoothies, and, of course, ferments! They come in all different shapes and sizes that you can use for brewing and storing. Although it's super convenient, please don't use plastic bottles or buckets for fermenting your beverages. They will leach chemicals into your brew, which you will then consume. There are some plastics that claim to be safe and free of dangerous chemicals like phthalates and bisphenol A, but for a material that is going to have an acidic drink inside it for a length of time, I just don't trust plastic. Stick to glass if you can. Metal of any kind is also a no-no. The acids will corrode the metal, which again ends up in your drink. Household stainless steel is also not ideal, as it only has a very thin coating and will corrode if it becomes scratched.

A Small Fine-Mesh Strainer

Most useful for kefir, this will also hold your little baby cauliflowers while you prepare their new home. Don't use a metal one, which may react with your brew; instead, use plastic.

A Regular Strainer or Sieve

My regular fine-mesh strainer is quite small, so I also have on hand a regular strainer, which I use mostly to strain out the fruits, herbs, or other flavorings from the second ferment of the beverage. But if you happen to have a larger fine-mesh strainer, that's really the only one you need.

Measuring Cups and Spoons

A definite must! I have used these measures in as many recipes as possible so that you don't continually have to use the scales for everything.

Cheesecloth

You will be able to find this at any kitchenware store or online. It doesn't need to be fancy, just with a tight enough weave to keep out any insects.

Funnel

A plastic funnel, although not absolutely essential, will save you a lot of unnecessary frustration, product loss, and sticky countertops.

Bottles

You will need some bottles for your finished products. I love the 1-liter bottles with the Grolsch-style swing-top caps. They keep your ferment airtight so that you will get a nice carbonation happening, and they look gorgeous for serving! You can find them at beer or wine supply shops or large housewares stores like Ikea. However, you can use anything you like. Again, I advocate glass bottles, with the caveat to just be sure to keep checking the pressure to prevent over-carbonation.

Labels or Masking Tape

Very useful! You think you will remember what's in that bottle, but it is so handy to have the date and ingredients clearly accessible.

I have split these frequently asked questions into sections on kombucha, kefir, and water kefir, but I hope you also will be able to find the answers to any questions you have relating to other ferments in this section.

Where do I get a SCOBY or kefir grains?

In a perfect world, you would have a generous fermenting friend who would share with you. However, if you are the pioneering fermenter in your group, there are other options, with online being the best resource. You can find anything online these days. There are some wonderful databases compiled of people in all different parts of the world willing to share their SCOBYs and grains with everyone, sometimes for free. A good Google search should set you in the right direction, but here are some suggestions.

Worldwide: The Kombucha Exchange: www.kombu.de; eBay: there are some wonderful sellers of SCOBYs and grains that you can find close to where you live.

USA and Canada: Cultures for Health: www.culturesforhealth.com.

Australia: Pink Farm: www.facebook.com/ourpinkfarm; the Weston A. Price Foundation (www.westonaprice.org) has a chapter in most parts of America and throughout many other countries. Check with the chapter leader in your area as to who has SCOBYs and grains to pass on.

KOMBUCHA FAQs

If there is mold on my SCOBY, is it still okay?

Mold can sometimes form on the surface of your SCOBY if you have slipped up somewhere along the line in keeping things clean. It will appear in small spots that are furry looking and either blue, green, or black. It looks like the mold that occurs on bread. If this happens to your SCOBY, unfortunately you have lost it. It is best to throw it out, or pop it on your compost pile, and start again.

My SCOBY has friends. Who are they?

If your SCOBY has stringy pieces of brown material that look like connective tissue hanging from it, believe it or not, this is good! These are strands of yeast. They can also hang out in little blobs. It's all good. SCOBYs have quite a personality. I often find myself talking to them when I check on their progress. I'm sure this helps! A SCOBY with hanging pieces of yeast everywhere and raised globs is a happy SCOBY. It may also develop bumps, holes, or jelly-like patches, and this is all fine. You don't want it to be perfectly plain and clean with no discoloration, as this is likely to mean it is inactive and therefore won't ferment the tea. The strains of yeast may also be seen moonlighting in the liquid, just floating around where they please. Or there may be a little party of them forming as sediment at the bottom of the jar. These are all normal by-products of the fermentation process.

Why is there is a cloudy haze on the surface of my kombucha?

Great! Don't touch it. After you add your SCOBY to your tea, move the jar to your chosen fermenting spot and leave it there undisturbed. This haze or almost oily-looking film on the surface is the beginning of the new mother. It usually begins to form around a couple of days into the brewing process, depending on the temperature of your home. If you move your jar and shake around the water, this process is disturbed and it will take longer to form again. Keep the jar as still as possible while your new SCOBY is growing.

Should a SCOBY sink or float?

The SCOBY may move around during the fermentation process. I find this so endearing, like a cat moving around in its basket to find the perfect comfortable position. Your SCOBY may float near the top, middle, or bottom, and it may move several times. It may be horizontal or vertical. If it does end up near the top, it may fuse with the newly forming mother. After fermentation has finished, you can separate the two by gently tearing them apart, or just use the newly fused supersize SCOBY for your next batch.

How do I know if it's working?

There are three main signs to look for in a successful kombucha.

First is the formation of a new mother on the surface of the liquid. Second is the development of yeast particles and stringy structures. And third, the liquid should taste slightly vinegary and less sweet than what you started with.

If none of this is happening, your mother may no longer be viable. The initial liquid may have been too warm when you added the SCOBY, which killed it, chlorinated water may be a problem, or perhaps it is too cold. Kombucha prefers a temperature of 75° to 85°F (24° to 30°C) for fermenting. You can purchase fancy kombucha-warming mats, or you can just wait patiently, as it will ferment eventually as long as the mother is viable. Back in the days when people would traditionally ferment kombucha, it was often in cold European conditions, so you may just need to be patient, as it will take a very long time—maybe up to a few months. As long as there is no mold, you're fine.

Something else to note is that cigarette smoke will damage the SCOBY, as will consistent smoke from an open fire, such as from a fireplace.

How sour should my kombucha be?

The level of acidity in your tea is important. That is what keeps the tea safe from mold and potential invading bacteria until the SCOBY produces enough acid of its own. The level of acidity can vary, and it depends on the sorts of tea and sugar you use, and also the health of your SCOBY. To maintain the perfect environment for your SCOBY, the kombucha should start with a pH lower than 4.6, and finish somewhere between 2.5 and 4.0.

The pH (potential hydrogen) is a measure for acidity. You may have heard of it in reference to the body, or in respect to gardening and soil composition. In this case, we are applying it to beverages. If you are interested in knowing the exact pH of your brew, you can purchase inexpensive pH testing strips from the local pharmacy. It really isn't necessary to test, though; as long as you have a slightly sour brew, you're on the right track.

What if I want a break from brewing?

Kombucha is quite robust compared to kefir. When you want to have a break from brewing, or if you want to store your extra SCOBYs, you can put them into hibernation. Place them in a clean glass jar, cover with brewed, unflavored kombucha tea, pop a lid on the jar, and keep in the refrigerator until you're ready to brew again. Walter Trupp of Trupps Cooking School in Melbourne, Australia (and fermenting aficionado), says he has kept his SCOBY this way for years and it has been fine.

What sort of tea is best?

Black tea is generally considered the best tea to use for kombucha brewing, but there are many others that you can use. The SCOBY uses not only the sugar to feed from, but also the tannins and polyphenols found in tea from the *Camellia sinensis* family. Green tea, white tea, and rooibos all work well. Pu-erh tea is a fermented Chinese variety of tea that is often recommended for use with kombucha. In pu-erh tea, the natural microbes living on the tea ferment the leaves. Yerba maté also makes a good substitute for black tea when making kombucha.

Herbal teas contain less (or sometimes none) of these properties of tannins or polyphenols. That is not to say that you cannot brew with herbal teas, but every couple of batches it is best to do a black tea brew to nourish the SCOBY again and keep it in optimal health. Alternatively, you can brew using part black tea and part herbal tea to help your SCOBY live to a ripe old age.

In terms of herbal teas, experimentation is the key. I recommend getting comfortable with brewing your kombucha first with the black tea and sugar combination. Once your confidence grows, along with your backup collection of SCOBYs, feel free to experiment with any tea you like. Keep in mind, though, that herbal teas containing volatile oils are thought to degrade and damage the SCOBY. Examples are peppermint, spearmint, rosemary, sage, and, to a lesser extent, chamomile. If you want to use these herbs with your brew, use them in the second fermentation so that you won't damage your precious SCOBY. Also, any herbal teas used should be organic.

What about the caffeine?

The caffeine that is left at the end of the fermentation process is very little. The fermentation process generally cuts the caffeine level by two-thirds. So, depending on what kind of tea you start with, you will have a different amount left. In his book *The Art of Fermentation*, Sandor Katz references a finished brew of black tea kombucha as containing 3.4 mg caffeine per 100 ml, which is far less than what is in a cup of black tea. In most people, this level of caffeine presents no problem. If, however, you have only to sniff a caramel macchiato and you're up all night, here are some strategies for reducing the caffeine content of your kombucha.

An old trick for reducing the caffeine in your cup of tea is to plunge your tea bag into a cup of hot water for about 30 seconds, then remove the tea bag, tip out the liquid, and start again with the same tea bag and fresh water. This process removes about half the caffeine from your finished drink.

Or use a mix of *Camellia sinesis* teas in your brew. Use black tea to make up only one-third of your mix, and use green or white tea for the rest, both of which are naturally lower in caffeine.

Last, incorporate herbal teas such as rooibos, which is caffeine-free and makes a lovely brew. Be sure to treat your SCOBY to some pure black tea after a couple of batches, though.

What about the sugar content?

The sugar in kombucha can put people off, but essentially it is there to feed your SCOBY, not to sweeten your drink. The website culturesforhealth.com says that there are 1 to 2 grams of sugar per 8 ounces (235 ml) of finished unflavored kombucha, which is a tiny amount.

What's up with that smell?

Your kombucha should smell slightly vinegary at the end of the fermentation process. The longer you leave it, the more vinegary-smelling it will become. If you notice any unpleasant smells, then this is a sign that your SCOBY is not well. Cheesy odors, rancid aromas, and eau de dirty socks are not normal, and if you smell anything like this, you should throw it out and begin again.

Help! Why isn't my kombucha bubbly?

One of my favorite things about kombucha—and there are many—is that you end up with a beautifully carbonated brew that is completely satisfying and refreshing. During the process of fermentation, the SCOBY forms a seal at the top of the jar, and the good bacteria and yeasts begin to consume the sugar in the tea, leaving the natural by-product of carbonation. If it is not bubbly, you may have let your kombucha brew for too long. Over-fermentation not only produces an extremely acidic, vinegary end product, but most of the good bacteria and yeasts will also die off, as they will have exhausted all their nourishment (the sugar).

To obtain a lovely, bubbly kombucha, don't let your first ferment get overly sour—just keep tasting it to test. Once you are happy with it, transfer it to a separate airtight bottle for the second fermentation with your chosen fruit, juice, or other flavoring. The yeasts will come to life and feast on the new sugars in the fruit, and thus create further carbonation for you.

KEFIR FAQS

What is the difference between kefir grains and kefir starter?

Kefir grains are the actual culture, whereas a kefir starter is a powdered product containing bacterial strains and whey powder. Kefir starter normally contains around seven or so different bacterial strains, whereas the kefir culture contains more than fifty. Kefir grains and starter can both be reused over time; however, the starter can be used only around five times before it becomes not viable.

Kefir starters can be useful for those just wanting to make the odd batch of kefir every now and then, as they are more convenient, but the kefir grains give a much better result in my experience—and are more fun!

What if I want to have a break from brewing my kefir?

You can give your kefir grains a little holiday in two ways. You can pop them into a small glass jar covered with a small amount of left-over brewed kefir and keep airtight in the refrigerator. Alternatively, you can dehydrate the grains by rinsing them thoroughly in filtered water and place them on a piece of unbleached

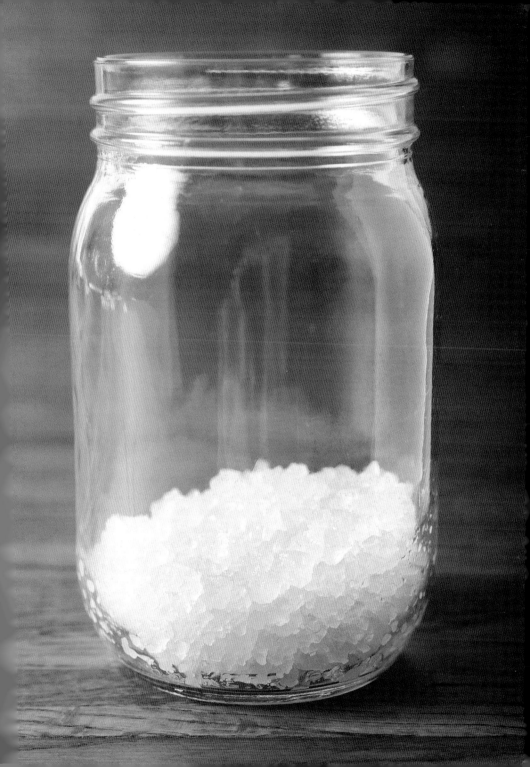

parchment or baking paper and dry at room temperature for three to five days or until completely dry. Store in an airtight jar in the fridge for around six months.

To rehydrate the grains again, treat them as you would any fresh batch of kefir, however, they may take two brews to regain their vigor again."

How can I tell if my milk is turning into kefir?

The milk will thicken to a drinking yogurt consistency and will taste more sour. It will also smell like a good-quality sour yogurt. You can adjust the sourness of your kefir by leaving it to ferment for a longer or shorter amount of time. If your kefir smells off, or tastes nasty, it is probably no good and you should not drink it.

What is kefir supposed to taste like?

Kefir can be an acquired taste. Although the taste varies depending on the length of fermentation, it does have a sour taste and is slightly effervescent. It is perfect for blending into smoothies or using in other recipes. A good idea if you are unsure may be to purchase some prepared kefir to taste-test it so that you will know what it is supposed to taste like, and whether you like it, before you invest the time into fermenting your own. Your homemade kefir will contain more good bacteria than store-bought varieties, and it is also much more cost-effective.

What types of milk can be used for culturing kefir?

You can use cow's, goat's, sheep's, or coconut milk. It is best to start off by culturing a few batches in cow's milk first, and then have a go at experimenting with different milks. I also advise that you return your grains to a dairy milk brew every second or third batch, to keep them happy and healthy.

Long-life and ultra-pasteurized milks are not recommended.

If you can get a hold of some nonhomogenized milk, you will notice the top layer of kefir will be a little more yellow in color, as the cream rises to the top.

The website culturesforhealth.com says that if you are using raw milk, you will need to wean your kefir grains onto it gradually. Make sure your grains are happy and pro-ducing good kefir, and then add a little raw milk into your next batch, then a little more for the following batch, and so on, until you have them in 100 percent raw milk. This is to give the grains time to establish their own bacteria before having to compete with those found in the raw milk.

My kefir has separated. What should I do?

This happens if you leave your kefir to culture for a longer time. Give it a good shake to form a nice smooth consistency. If the result is too sour for you, ferment it for a shorter time frame next time. You can also try culturing your milk using a ratio of fewer grains to more milk to reduce the strength. It's just a matter of playing around until you find something that suits you.

WATER KEFIR (TIBICOS) FAQS

My grains have disappeared! What happened?

This can sometimes happen if you do not feed your water kefir regularly, as tibicos is a little moodier than the milk variety. If you don't keep up the regular feeding, the grains can disintegrate in the sour ferment created due to the acidity. If this happens, unfortunately your tibicos are gone forever, and you will need to start again with new ones. You will know if your water kefir is not happy, as it will not ferment the sugar water, and the mix will stay sweet.

Why aren't my grains growing/multiplying?

Water kefir is certainly moodier than milk kefir grains or kombucha, or any other ferment, really. They are sensitive in that you need to feed them frequently, and if you don't, they will punish you by not fermenting your beverage. If your water kefir is not growing, this may be because you have left your grains for too long and they are literally starving! The upside to that is that the turnaround time of the finished brew is also much faster.

Your grains may also suffer from extreme temperatures. If they are not growing, they may not be viable anymore. They may, however, just not be growing but still be capable of producing good kefir. If this is the case, I like to romance them with a dried organic fig and a little molasses added into the normal sugar water to see if I can coax them to grow. If you are not sure whether they are still good, keep culturing your kefir, and if you get a product that smells off or rancid, they are no good. Throw it all out and find another lot of grains.

ACKNOWLEDGMENTS

To my wonderful husband, Mat: Thank you for your love, patience, support, advice, and tolerance of having a million jars of fermented goodness all over the house. I am so grateful for your inspiration and encouragement to believe in myself, and for the endless cups of tea! You are fabulous, and I love you very much.

To Ivy: You are a daily source of wonder and entertainment. Thank you for making my heart so happy and for reminding me what is important. I love you!

There are several special people who have gone out of their way to help, advise, and encourage this book along:

Thank you to Jo, for always being interested, asking the right questions, and encouraging me to elaborate on my ideas. You are wonderful.

Thank you to Miin, for your generous contribution of experience and knowledge.

Thank you to Emma, for your undying support of all my projects, and of my life in general. You are amazing, and I love you!

Thank you to Suzie, for withstanding numerous long discussions at all times of day and for always being in my corner. I love you!

And to my wonderful family and everyone else who has supported this project along the way: Thank you so much!

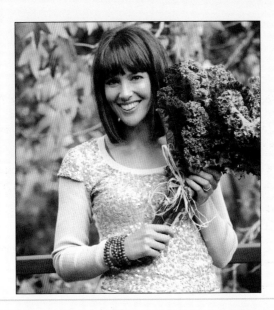

Meg Thompson is a practicing naturopath, cook, mother, whole foods blogger, businesswoman, and health advocate who lives in Melbourne, Australia.

Meg's interest in health, food, and the role of food as medicine has shaped her career and lifestyle. Following an early career in psychology and education, Meg completed studies in naturopathy, nutrition, and herbal medicine and now runs a successful clinical practice where she specializes in digestive, women's, and children's health.

As her practice grew, Meg gradually became inundated by patients who either had become disconnected from food and its role in maintaining health and preventing disease or had struggled to overcome food allergies and lifestyle-induced illnesses. Finding that most of her clinical practice centered on educating patients on the benefits of a diet diverse in fresh and whole foods, Meg sought to share her views and passion with a larger audience through her blog, www.mywholefoodromance.com.

Meg's research and writings have regularly affirmed the value of ancient food preparations, such as fermentation, on health. Using her own home as a laboratory, Meg experimented with the exotic and often eccentric range of fermented cultures and colonies and discovered that it was easy to create foods that support digestion, immunity, and well-being through fermentation, returning essential bacteria and enzymes to her family's diet.

This book represents that research, and Meg's journey.

INDEX